# Nicotine:
# The Drug That Never Was

# Nicotine:
# The Drug That Never Was

## Volume II:

## A Change of Mind

by

Chris Holmes

Copyright © 2010 by Chris Holmes

All rights reserved. No part of this book may be reproduced, stored, or transmitted by any means—whether auditory, graphic, mechanical, or electronic—without written permission of both publisher and author, except in the case of brief excerpts used in critical articles and reviews. Unauthorized reproduction of any part of this work is illegal and is punishable by law.

ISBN: 978-1-4461-6148-7

# Contents

| | | |
|---|---|---|
| Introduction | | 1 |
| Section Eleven | The Beliefs and Suggestions that Support the Tobacco Habit | 9 |
| Section Twelve | The Willpower Myth | 87 |
| Section Thirteen | Why Doctors Do Not Provide Hypnotherapy | 115 |
| Section Fourteen | Those Two Imposters: Success and Failure | 163 |
| Section Fifteen | The Art of Hypnotherapy in Practice | 193 |
| Section Sixteen | Stage Hypnosis (part 2) | 227 |
| Section Seventeen | Hypnotherapy v. Science | 289 |
| Appendix | | 321 |

# Introduction

i). First of all, a hearty welcome back to all those who read Volume I and were curious enough to investigate this second part also. Really it is just the latter half of the same book - the damn thing was getting a bit too big for anyone to lug around, so I hacked it in two. If you haven't read Volume I, and are curious as to what it was all about, a copy of the contents pages are included at the back of this book as an appendix.

In Volume I, most of the emphasis was on destroying the myth of nicotine addiction - identifying nicotine as a poison, not a drug - and defining the Compulsive Habit as distinct from addiction. The single most useful aspect of all that, for practical purposes in therapy, is for us to be able to recognise that cravings are not withdrawal symptoms and are not connected to nicotine in any way. The truth is, humans commonly experience all sorts of cravings, they are not all about tobacco and indeed some do not involve any substance, such as the urge felt by the compulsive gambler to put £50 to win on *Nowhere To Run* in the 3.50 race at Haydock Park. Nor is a craving signal truly a desire or a need, although it can certainly *feel* like either, as a subjective experience. It is actually an impulse originating from the brain, prompting a certain action or behaviour which we may then regard as spontaneous, or just habitual.

Of course, we are able to mentally attach the notion that this truly is a need or a desire, and that might then *seem* utterly convincing. Such notions may also disintegrate at some time, without the behaviour necessarily ceasing, as in the perception: "These days I just seem to be smoking for the sake of it", or "I don't know why I'm eating this, I don't even want it really". Pleasure may or may not be perceived to be a factor but if it is, this aspect obviously needs addressing in the proposal for positive change. Yet the impulse itself is a physical urge to act - quite distinct from those other, attached mental notions – and is deliberately fired off by the Subconscious mind. Just as easily as the Subconscious can trigger this impulse, it can transfer it to something else or eliminate it altogether. It can also alter any beliefs or emotions that may support the behaviour too, upon request, during a hypnotherapy session. It doesn't have to though, so the role of the therapist is not to instruct the Subconscious mind but is really a combination of advocate and diplomat.

The Subconscious mind can choose to change any of these things, either during a therapy session or sometime afterward, regardless of whether the conscious mind believes this is possible or not. Usually the conscious mind of the client does not expect that change is going to happen, and is very surprised when it does, not least because the conscious mind didn't do anything at all during the therapy and didn't really believe in the Subconscious anyway, except perhaps in theory. (This conscious skepticism is not universal, but is very common at this point in history.) However, the Subconscious may alternatively ignore the request to make a change: or only partly change it, change it sometime later on or only change it temporarily.

Cynics will often leap on this sort of initial outcome, as if it demonstrated that hypnosis 'doesn't work', 'doesn't last' or 'wears off', when really it is simply that the Subconscious does what it likes when it chooses and may not respond wholeheartedly right away. Relapse isn't failure unless you interpret it as such, and hesitation is a very different thing from refusal. Permanent change can usually be established anyway with more time spent on the issue – but only if the client chooses to pursue it. Some choose to walk away, wrongly assuming that if 'it' didn't 'work' immediately, then 'it failed' so why pursue it? That lame attitude rarely wins success in *any* endeavour, but there's a lot of it about. As a friend of mine used to say, that's not the attitude that made Britain Great! Persistence is the key to success in many things, and sometimes it is required in the hypnotherapy process too.

This Volume is mainly about the beliefs that commonly support the habit, and many other incorrect notions which we routinely change with hypnotherapy – one of which is that hypnotherapy is a load of mumbo-jumbo and it won't work. This is quite a common piece of ignorance, but not everyone holds that belief. Beliefs are simply ideas that you have ceased to question for the time being, and they are not set in stone. Some are more firmly held than others. In fact, our beliefs naturally change a good deal during the course of a lifetime. We don't believe the same things from one end of our lives to the other, because of course we live and learn. Some learn a lot more than they live, some live a lot more than they learn... most of us just get a little wiser every year and try not to take it all too seriously.

I think it is helpful to remind ourselves, periodically, that we are all just glorified monkeys at the end of the day. It explains the monkey business.

Monkey see, monkey do. After all, that's how we all started smoking, isn't it?

ii). The tobacco story has so many curious twists and turns that I am never really surprised when another one pops up. In Volume One I mentioned that I hadn't quite managed to discover exactly when the "nicotine addiction" story started, as an interpretation of compulsive use and I suggested that if anyone was intrigued about that then they should keep digging and if they found anything enlightening to let me know. This inspired Chepstowbased hypnotherapist Marc Bishop to investigate further and he contacted me recently to tell me about Lennox Johnston, of whom I had never heard.

The fact that I had never heard of him is interesting in itself, because it turns out that Lennox Johnston – and be honest, you've never heard of him either, right? - was the first person to use nicotine in isolation to offset the impulse to reach for tobacco. In other words he invented Nicotine Replacement Therapy (NRT) – the very thing my book denounces. Now, NRT is prescribed and sold all over the world, so if we all know about innovators like Alexander Fleming and Louis Pasteur, how come Lennox Johnston is never mentioned when people talk about NRT?

Actually it is probably because he was rather like me: he made a bit of a nuisance of himself and everybody felt quite certain that he was wrong... which causes me to feel a certain, odd kinship with the chappie even though he is very much my adversary in this argument, for am I not in a very similar position here, trying to explain why smoking is not what most people presently think it is? Here is an extract from Johnston's typical pronouncements to the editor of *The Lancet* circa 1953:

> "I think it more sensible and scientifically satisfying to recognise tobacco-smoking as a drug addiction from start to finish. It varies in degree from slight to serious. The euphemism "habit" should be discarded completely... no smoker derives positive pleasure and benefit from tobacco. The bliss of headache or toothache relieved is analogous to that of craving for tobacco appeased."

Reading that, one is immediately reminded of Allen Carr's later observations in *The Easy Way To Stop Smoking*. The final point is overstated – rather like Carr's analogy for craving-relief, which was the bliss of removing a tight shoe. But what all three of us would agree upon is that the 'pleasure' of lighting up is not really a pleasure but a relief: the cessation of an irritation. Carr and Johnston both interpret this as evidence of addiction because they are reminded of the 'withdrawal symptom' experienced by heroin addicts. Although Carr describes arriving at this conclusion as if it were a moment of inspirational genius, it is obvious from reading this snippet penned by Johnston about three decades earlier that *Easy Way* was not quite as original as Allen Carr seemed to think it was! His interpretation of the smoking problem clearly has its origins here in Lennox Johnston's view, although I doubt Carr had ever heard of him either. He certainly never mentioned him in any of his own writings to my knowledge.

So what did the medical profession think of Johnston's insistence that tobacco smoking was a drug addiction in the 1950's? Well, we have managed to find this frank repudiation by none other than the Honorary Secretary of the Society for the Study of Addiction, one H. Pullar-Strecker, in response to Johnston's assertions:

> "Much as one may 'crave' for one's smoke, tobacco is no drug of addiction. Proper addicts... will stop at nothing to obtain the drug that their system demands imperatively."

Smokers often tell me that they are puzzled by the fact that although they wouldn't normally go for nine hours without a cigarette during the day, when they are on a plane it doesn't seem to bother them until they land, or very shortly before they land. The only exceptions seem to be smokers who resent the restriction, or have a problem with flying anyway. Likewise we hear of smokers seemingly untroubled by cravings during a spell in hospital, or more ordinarily whenever they go anywhere where smoking is commonly accepted as being out of the question, such as *Mothercare* or the Finsbury Park Mosque. It seems that as long as the smoker accepts that restriction, there will be no urge to smoke until they leave that situation. That is certainly not withdrawal, and falling nicotine levels in the body during the nine-hour flight (for example) are clearly irrelevant. The "nicotine receptors" in the brain are hardly in a position to appreciate the smoking ban on aircraft – or observe it – so this certainly begs the question "Why are they not 'going crazy' - as the NRT advert would have us believe is the cause of smokers' cravings – in all of the situations mentioned above?" For of course Pullar-Strecker was right: the heroin addict cannot do that. If a heroin addict gets on a plane and the heroin level in the blood falls low *then they are ill,* it doesn't matter what they are doing or where they are situated. *That's* withdrawal.

Lennox Johnston was a Glaswegian GP who had been a smoker himself and according to his obituary in the *British Medical Journal* (Volume 292, dated 29/03/86) he quit smoking twice. It relates how he pondered his compulsion to continue smoking and "wondered what would be the effect of stopping" – only to find that it proved easier than he expected. A year or so later, he started smoking again and after that it took him "two agonising years" to give up.

Later he became an anti-smoking campaigner and began to experiment with pure solutions of nicotine which he often administered to himself, once with near-fatal consequences. He also wrote to *The Lancet* describing an experiment he devised himself which involved about thirty smokers who apparently allowed him to inject them with nicotine whenever they felt the urge to reach for tobacco, which Johnston claimed then subsided. Although this certainly does not qualify as a bona fide clinical trial, it can be regarded as the first ever attempt to trial nicotine replacement as a concept. *The Lancet* published Johnston's letter, and so began the biggest medical mistake of the 20$^{th}$ Century – though of course, everyone thought he was wrong at the time.

Well – not quite everyone. Throughout the history of tobacco-smoking in Europe there have been occasional voices calling it an "addiction", though quite what those individuals thought that term really meant is not easy to determine now. Yet for most of that history nearly everybody simply regarded it as a filthy habit – which is pretty accurate. A complex compulsive habit to be exact – for a full definition of that see Chapter Ten in Volume One, where I spell out the key differences between that and true drug addiction.

It is only very recently, in fact, that the "nicotine addiction" interpretation has become the general impression and not everyone believes it even now. There have always been voices in the scientific community who have pointed out the inconsistencies but they couldn't explain the compulsive element because they didn't have the key knowledge of the normal operations of the human Subconscious mind and how it organises and activates compulsive habitual behaviour. So they got shouted down – as did the tobacco companies who tried to point out that other habitual behaviours that did not involve any substances – such as shopaholics and compulsive gamblers – seemed to be of a similar order, but eventually they too accepted the new doctrine and dropped the argument. Not because the argument was invalid, but because they were pretty much on their own at that point. The anti-smokers were on a roll and have been ever since.

Factually the tobacco companies were right - but because smoking is damaging to health they didn't have a chance of getting their point heard as the scientific proof of real harm emerged during the 1960s and has continued to be the justification for everything that has changed since. Every anti-smoking policy or restriction that has been introduced from that time onwards has been justified with a reminder of the enormous harm that tobacco does to human health. Real enquiry became irrelevant in the rush to condemn, and any persons raising queries about the addiction tale began to sound like apologists for the tobacco industry. To some extent this is still the case today, the only difference being that the nicotine tale is now supporting a completely new industry. Or rather, two: the "therapeutic nicotine" industry, and the medical side of the smoking cessation industry which in some countries is now funded by the public purse, pouring millions into the coffers of the drug companies involved and getting nothing in return but a useless poison!

It's a pity it never occurred to Lennox Johnston to wonder why he found it surprisingly easy to quit the first time, but it took "two agonising years" the second time. Surely the role of nicotine was the same in both cases and what that gives us straight away is the clue that nicotine isn't the difficulty: the perception of 'ease' or 'difficulty' – even 'agony' – results from other variables that are nothing to do with the contents of the cigarette. That's why expert hypnotherapy can usually resolve the matter on a single occasion by dealing with those factors, whereas NRT does not.

The medical establishment thought Johnston was wrong, in fact they ignored him for years and don't even talk about him now. The tobacco companies thought it was just a habit, as did virtually all smokers at the time. Some still do, despite all the crazy nicotine propaganda that is really just marketing for NRT dressed up as medical orthodoxy.

The irony is that the medical establishment were in fact quite correct in the first place. So it may now seem to many people as if I'm the mad eccentric, when all I'm pointing out is exactly what everyone knew anyway before Lennox Johnston came along. If they had only stuck to their initial assessment that *he* was the mad eccentric, then they could have remained quite correct all along and we could have avoided this crazy detour around and around and around the poison nicotine, which is not the real reason people struggle to quit through their own efforts, as I explained in Volume One.

Lennox Johnston lived until he was 86, surviving long enough to see his initially unpopular pronouncements adopted as the standard medical view. By mistake.

# Section Eleven

## The Beliefs and Suggestions that Support the Tobacco Habit

### *including* Smoking and Self-Harm: a parallel

As I described in the last section of Volume I, some compulsive habits have ideas or beliefs attached to them which may become part of the problem. In this section I will list the common ideas that may become attached to the useless activity of smoking tobacco, and also how to get rid of them. I must emphasize that these ideas must be challenged on a conscious *and* Subconscious level, or they can cause relapse later if they have not been adequately addressed in each mental arena separately. Relapse is still *possible* later on, but it is much less likely if these ideas and beliefs no longer hold at any level.

First, a list:

a. I enjoy smoking, it's a pleasure.
b. I'm hooked. I am addicted, that's why I can't stop doing it.

c. It is very hard to stop smoking, everybody says so.
d. It relaxes me.
e. It helps me deal with stress.
f. It helps me concentrate at work.
g. It helps me keep my weight down.
h. It alleviates boredom, gives me something to do with my hands.
i. It is very nice to have one after a meal.
j. It just goes together with a drink, doesn't it?
k. I only smoke a bit.
l. I'll be alright, it won't happen to me.
m. I don't want to stop smoking.

If you ask habitual smokers why they smoke, they may say all sorts of things including some of the statements listed above, which are the most common responses. Few smokers will believe *all* of those things, but most will believe some of them or else recognise that they once did believe things like that. Beliefs often change anyway over time, and of course this is all very subjective. But just to make it a bit more complex, these beliefs may be operating on a conscious *or* Subconscious level in any one person. Thus a smoker may recognise logically, on a conscious level that nicotine has no relaxing qualities, yet still *feel* that smoking helps them relax, because their Subconscious has some other impression which has never been challenged at that mental level.

This fact – that we hold beliefs, or have ideas influencing our choices and behaviour at two different levels – represents a major problem with approaches like counselling and psychotherapy. There is only one way to challenge Subconscious beliefs, and that is to talk to the Subconscious about it. If a therapist is not doing that, then change is limited to conscious attitudes most of the time. You might go on doing that for ten sessions, until the client is very annoyed and frustrated, with the impression that you are only telling them what they know (consciously) already, but it hasn't changed the way they *feel,* which is entirely to do with their Subconscious attitude. If they were never in trance during any of that, their Subconscious wasn't even listening to those conversations.

During discussions about tobacco, smokers may well mention the real reason they smoke – habit – but most of them do not realise that this is the only *real* reason. If people smoke for long enough, however, they will usually have come to that conclusion in the end. When I am working with clients aged in their sixties or seventies and I ask them why they smoke, most of them will simply say "Habit". They tend not to offer any of those other ideas on the list, because by that time in their lives they have come to recognise that smoking is just meaningless, pointless repetition of the same thing every day.

Part of the reason these other ideas and beliefs exist is because we have all been led to believe that our decisions, choices and behaviour are simply a matter of freewill. So we then have to try to justify our actual behaviour with a plausible 'reason' generated on a conscious level, to maintain the illusion of conscious choice. We don't have to look far for the plausible 'reasons' because we were listening to the previous generation repeatedly declaring them all the time we were growing up. So they are in fact drilled into us, and whether we seriously regard them as logical or not, the ideas remain 'useful' - something we can tell ourselves or other people if we feel a need to justify our smoking behaviour. Non-smokers too sometimes refer to these notions and beliefs when commenting upon the behaviour of smokers, as if everybody 'knows' these things to be true, because the ideas are universally familiar. That does not mean they are true.

Some of these ideas, since they are mentioned repeatedly throughout our development, inevitably become established on a Subconscious level. The other huge influence on the Subconscious was tobacco advertising and promotion. This has now been banned in the U.K., but the last few generations were absolutely bombarded with millions of suggestions and images that were carefully crafted and designed to encourage a positive attitude towards tobacco. Advertising is a form of hypnosis most of the time. Very little of it is aimed at the conscious mind, so it does not influence the conscious mind much at all, which therefore tends to dismiss advertising, as if it were just a pathetic attempt to influence other, less intelligent people! Some advertising actually appears like that on purpose, playing up to the conscious mind's assumption whilst still getting the message across to the Subconscious, despite the irritation and contempt of the conscious mind. There are lots of ways of getting noticed, and being irritating unfortunately works quite well.

There are a few exceptions to this, in which the conscious mind is the target of the suggestion, such as when a brand of tobacco is being advertised on the basis of low price alone. The Subconscious is not motivated by ideas like 'value for money', that is the analytical mind's concern. But the vast majority of tobacco promotion in the past was much more imaginative than that.

Due to the gradual increase in restrictions over the years, regarding the unsuitability of this suggestion or that, tobacco advertising went through a bizarre series of changes over those generations. "You're never alone with a Strand" is one laughable suggestion that many remember from many years ago. "Happiness is a cigar called Hamlet" was a very long-running campaign slogan, and those adverts were regularly on television when I was growing up. Many of them featured a short cartoon scenario which depicted a frustrating situation in which a hapless character repeatedly failed to succeed in some task, such as trying to get a golf ball out of a bunker. With each attempt, tension mounted as we were invited to identify with the character's predicament, reminding us of how we feel when things just will not go right no matter what we do. Suddenly he stops trying (relief!), there is the sound of a match striking (suggesting the lighting of a cigar) and immediately there is relaxing classical music and a plume of smoke drifts lazily upwards (we are rising above the problem – floating - at ease once more). The fact that it is really the music that relaxes the viewer can easily be missed in a visual medium, as we are more immediately aware of the images, which are suggesting that tobacco should get the credit for the fact that peace has returned.

In reality it goes like this: first, the annoying scenario was designed to deliberately wind us up, then there was relief when it stopped, followed instantly by very relaxing music – none of which is connected to tobacco in any way. Even if the cartoon character were a real smoker, all that would have already happened before any of the chemicals in the smoke reached the bloodstream. It is a clever trick, but completely dishonest because there is nothing in tobacco smoke that makes people relax – quite the reverse. And if you flatter yourself that none of that kind of deception had any effect upon *your* view of tobacco, just bear in mind that is only your conscious view. If you ever heard anyone say something like this:

> "Yes, and he was so upset he needed a cigarette to calm himself down..."

... and you accepted that as if it was true, then the tobacco companies didn't spend millions of pounds every year doing that for nothing. Even if you don't smoke yourself, if you are prepared to accept the idea that others might genuinely need or 'use' cigarettes purposely, or that smoking tobacco truly calms a person down, then it went in. The conscious mind may recognise the suggestion for what it is, or it may not. Yet it still got in 'under the radar' as it were – all of which accounts for this common exchange in the first part of a smoking session:

> Therapist: Do you feel as if tobacco has helped you in any way, with the ups and downs of everyday life?
> 
> Client (frowning): Well... I know it doesn't *really*... (conscious belief based upon facts learned) ...but sometimes... I just *feel as if* it does,

even though I know that's rubbish really. Still, whenever I get stressed that's the first thing I'll do – reach for a cigarette.

That *feeling* is based upon the Subconscious impression that tobacco is calming or relaxing, a direct result of the decades of tobacco promotion which incessantly repeated that suggestion. Notice how this demonstrates that we can be holding opposing views at the same time on different levels. One does not cancel out the other because they are not colliding, as they are operating in different mental circuits. The Subconscious view is supporting the habit pattern, as if it is not simply repeating it but doing so for a reason. The fact that the conscious mind knows the reason is false makes no difference, because the Subconscious knows nothing about that. That knowledge was picked up by the conscious mind at some point, operating on another level altogether. The smoker is only really aware of the general feeling that smoking 'should help', the factual observation that they feel an impulse to reach for tobacco when stress builds up, which they may well mistake for a 'need'... and the confusing fact that they also know this is not really doing anything useful, so their behaviour seems to be at odds with their knowledge. All of which is perfectly understandable once you let go of the idea that the conscious mind directs all our behaviour and choices. It obviously does not.

## What are you Suggesting?

One elderly client told me that when he first started work there was a poster on the wall of the canteen which featured an astonishing suggestion. He could no longer remember the tobacco brand, but let's say for the sake of argument it was Black Cat. The poster said: "Now have a Black Cat and *digest* that sandwich!" What a difference there is between that kind of blatant bullshit and the obscure, almost mystical imagery of the poster campaigns that we ended up with just before tobacco advertising was finally outlawed in the UK. I remember looking at one billboard that simply showed a lonely, ancient gas pump and a lot of empty desert (Marlboro?) and thinking: "What on earth are they trying to say to me?" I like to think I'm pretty good with suggestion, but I seriously doubt that image would influence anyone with regard to product or brand, except perhaps to put them off a bit.

But that was the endgame. It got weird, as things often do just before the axe falls, but for most of the twentieth century tobacco firms had it all their own way because of the vast sums of money they could fling around, rather like the pharmaceutical companies today. Advertisers were falling over themselves to win contracts with Big Tobacco, because those were the easiest adverts of the lot – all you had to do was show people relaxing, laughing, socialising, drinking and smoking, and slap the brand-name clearly across it, and there you go! Smoking is seen to be pleasurable and relaxing, smokers are popular and stylish with a devil-may-care outlook that others apparently warm to, and they're all out having a wonderful time.

By the time it was finally ended, the damage had already been done: we had all been brainwashed into believing that tobacco actually had a use or was pleasurable in some way, and once that idea is established in the Subconscious mind it will continue to influence behaviour and spontaneous responses indefinitely – long after the adverts themselves have disappeared. The periodic scare campaigns by government or health organisations are unlikely to remedy that situation because they are nowhere near as sustained, and do not challenge the original suggestions anyway, so the main ideas I listed at the start of this section are allowed to remain in play.

Actually there is not a shred of truth in any of those statements on the list, and I am not the first to say so either. Several other writers and therapists have pointed these things out before, most notably Allen Carr. But what many of these commentators failed to understand is that in order to solve the smoking problem easily it would not normally be enough just to point out these falsehoods to the conscious mind alone. Both mental departments need the full explanation of the reality if we are going to get the habit shut down *and* prevent relapse in the majority of cases.

In hypnotherapy cases where relapse into smoking occurs, it is very likely that this aspect of the therapy has been neglected, conducted inadequately or simply not yet accepted by the client. At one time – when smoking was still allowed in theatres - stage hypnotists often used to ask a smoker to come up on stage and simple aversion techniques would be advanced, by direct suggestion, to demonstrate dramatic changes to a smoker's immediate reaction to smoke. Smokers probably imagine that this is how a hypnotherapist would go about it too, as if that will stop somebody from ever smoking again. By itself, that approach is unlikely to have long-term effect - it just creates an immediate but temporary aversion to tobacco smoke. Since that smoker still has the same beliefs and ideas about smoking that supported the original habit, they will almost certainly revert to the original habit in due course. On the stage, the smoking volunteer probably only accepted the aversion suggestion for the purposes of the demonstration anyway, it was just a bit of drama for entertainment purposes, so that would usually be the limit of their response. Similar relapses after hypnotherapy are more likely to happen if the supporting beliefs and ideas are allowed to maintain. If we want permanent change then we have to be thorough.

What follows is a summary of what I say to clients about these 'reasons' for smoking, but please note that in a real stop smoking session these points are made a number of times during the session. In the pre-talk I make sure I have acceptance of the logical truth of it on a conscious level, and then during the trance section I will make these points again in a number of different ways, to make sure the Subconscious is fully up to speed with that as well. To neglect this is to risk non-acceptance of the change, or later relapse. As I have mentioned elsewhere, this is the reason self-help books on smoking may not achieve lasting change either, even if they are making the same points. Reading a self-help book is a critical, analytical process, which means the reader is not in trance, so the Subconscious will not be picking up the information that way, even if the conscious mind can appreciate the logic of it.

If the author has some basic insight that the Subconscious mind needs information too, sometimes a CD is included with a self-help book, which (it is supposed) will provide for that, and the reader is instructed to listen whilst relaxing comfortably with eyes closed. Unfortunately, the listener cannot ask any questions, isn't told how to respond positively and – crucially – is not warned in advance that it might well seem, to the conscious mind, as if nothing useful is happening at all. As a result of these omissions, the listener will probably assume nothing *is* happening, and this will result in a flat or negative mood, with negative results. This is not an example of hypnotherapy failing, it is a very common example of a poor substitute not being up to the job. There was no real hypnotherapy involved.

Now it is time to take each one of the smokers' responses on the list, and explain how a therapist can demonstrate that it is a misunderstanding.

### a). "I enjoy smoking, it's a pleasure."

Not all smokers believe they enjoy smoking. Even the ones that do didn't always believe it. And just because you believe that something is a pleasure does not mean it is. It can just *seem* that way, at times – and for good reasons.

Is tobacco smoking a pleasure? Very early on in a smoking session I will test the client's view on this. What I actually ask them is: "Do you feel as if you enjoy smoking?" These are the typical answers:

"No, I hate it!"
"No, not anymore... I used to."

"I only enjoy the odd one... the rest I'm just smoking for the sake of it."

"I enjoy some of them."

"I suppose I must like it. Otherwise I wouldn't do it, would I?"

"Yes, I really do enjoy smoking."

"Oh, definitely – I love my cigarettes!"

The second and third answers on the above list are the most common ones we hear as hypnotherapists, as you might expect from people who have decided to have therapy to stop smoking. But this wide range of responses would appear to indicate that tobacco smoking is a very subjective experience. However, these differences vanish when I ask about the client's first ever smoking experience:

> "Oh, God it was awful! I was nearly sick, and I coughed and spluttered, it was embarrassing really. God knows why I tried it again! Just stupid, I suppose..."

Of course there is always one client who has to be different, and claim – rather proudly, for some bizarre reason – that they never coughed at all, and took to it immediately like a duck to water. They are either lying because they have a compulsive habit of being contrary, or are just anatomically weird. We are not supposed to inhale anything that is not air, so if we attempt to inhale smoke we naturally come up against a barrier. The smoke is instantly detected by the Subconscious: *That is not air!* Inhaling smoke is not only very unpleasant, it is almost impossible to do at first. Smoke is not supposed to get into the lungs. It causes damage, and pollutants from the smoke can get into the bloodstream. It is dangerous to our survival, so there are defences in place to protect us from the consequences of doing something that risky.

The first time we attempt to inhale smoke, reflexes are kicked in instantly by the Subconscious to protect the body: coughing, choking and perhaps even retching in some cases. Reflexes are immediate muscular contractions that can protect us from all kinds of hazards, like touching a hot surface for example. They are operated instantaneously by the Subconscious mind, and indeed have usually already happened before the conscious mind has even registered what occurred and why. The conscious mind has little or no control over reflexes, and the reflex will normally overrule conscious intention, if it conflicts with that defensive reaction. So the coughing reflex is the Subconscious mind's first comment on the whole idea. You just inhaled toxic fumes! It kicks them back with some force.

This is not pleasant. Whatever makes us feel inclined to pick up the second cigarette, it certainly isn't because the first one was delightful. On the contrary, smokers are quick to acknowledge that the first cigarette made them feel dizzy and sick. So I point out to them, "If you later came to believe you were enjoying that experience, what changed was *your perception of it.* Smoke didn't change a bit. What we really do during the hypnotherapy process is change your perception back to what it was initially, because you were right in the first place. Smoke is unpleasant, and so is the effect of inhaling it!"

But the *idea* that smoking is a pleasure – the suggestion - was thoroughly drilled into all of us long before we ever tried to smoke that first foul cigarette. Throughout childhood, we were all exposed to thousands of suggestions that smoking is a luxury or a pleasure, mainly through advertising of course, but also because of the way smokers themselves talk about smoking, and the way they 'act it out' – as if smoking were a relief, a pleasure or a kind of 'freedom' to indulge themselves – which is a direct result of the tobacco industries' suggestions, even though the smoker does not usually realise that.

In truth we can trace this idea back still further: even before we are old enough to understand advertising, we make an assumption about tobacco. When we are very small and first making sense of the world around us – putting things in categories in the mind – we notice adults smoking. Now to a little child, this is very straightforward: children must do as they are told, but adults can do what they like. So if an adult is smoking, apparently voluntarily, the child assumes they must *like* it. It must be pleasant. Nothing else would make sense to a young child.

Some adults even allow the young child to sample the cigarette or pipe at some point, either to amuse themselves or perhaps in the hope it will put the child off forever. Of course the child instantly perceives that the smoke is nasty and disgusting, which it is. This might be surprising to the child, but only a little. Already in that young mind the recognition that kids' stuff and grown-ups' stuff can be radically different will be forming. Grown-ups eat things kids don't like, watch very boring TV programmes, have conversations the child cannot relate to. They don't even play out with their friends, for God's sake. Instead they all sit around smoking, drinking horrible drinks and having stupid boring conversations, they never have any fun. Adult choices and preferences are a continual mystery to children, so when grown-ups consume things that smell disgusting or breathe smoke in and out, this just matches every other bit of alien adult weirdness the child is getting used to.

Nevertheless, the assumption is established that the adult must in the end be doing that because they like it. Now, add to that all of the tobacco advertising to which the young mind is subjected over many years. Thousands of images and slogans hammering the idea home: It's a pleasure! It's a luxury! It's a wonderful thing. "Happiness is a cigar called Hamlet!" as they used to be allowed to say on the telly. Tobacco advertising has now finally been banned in the U.K. but smokers everywhere were subjected to many thousands of adverts like that, all the time they were growing up.

In ordinary life, suggestion has its effect in this way: if you hear something once or twice, it doesn't make much impression. But if you hear the same message day in, day out, over many years, it makes a very deep impression in the Subconscious mind. That is why tobacco manufacturers spent so much money repeating those messages every year until the adverts were finally made illegal. It is called mental conditioning, and works so well it can even convince non-smokers. Ask a person who never developed a smoking habit why other people smoke, and they might well say they do it for pleasure, they like doing it – even though they know from their own personal experience, many of them, that the reason they're a non-smoker is because they found the experience too revolting to bear.

Actually, only certain types of advert are mental conditioning. To be more accurate, we could regard advertising as:

a. <u>Straightforward Promotion</u> when it is undeniably true, as in "New Squidburgers - only £1.99 at Tesco!"
b. <u>Mental Conditioning</u> when it is only plausible or arguably true, but really a matter of opinion, as in: "Love your feet - buy the foot powder fungus is most afraid of: HappyToes!"
c. <u>Brainwashing</u> when it is certainly untrue, like the suggestion that a cigarette helps you to digest food, or that old coffee billboard campaign "Rise – Shine" which suggested that we cannot expect to achieve a state of true wakefulness unless we drink some Nescafe.

If you always start the day with a coffee yourself, you may be thinking: "No, hang on - that's true, isn't it?" Yes, as evidenced by the fact that all the folk who never touch the stuff keep falling helplessly back to sleep, always set off late for work, crash the car, forget to feed the baby, can't hold down a job. Why doesn't somebody tell them? The brain cannot function properly without Nescafe, it's just a fact. It is a curious anomaly in our evolution as a species.

On the other hand, perhaps the nice people at Nescafe can explain why, despite drinking loads of coffee, I had all those problems anyway? Come to think of it, since I stopped drinking coffee altogether I don't seem to have had any accidents or bad luck. Nor have I been attacked in the street, not once! It could just be a coincidence, I don't know - but if you've been plagued by any problems like that, try cutting out the coffee and see if that helps. That's my little health tip for today.

## Back to Tobacco

The effect of all this advertising-suggestion programmes us so effectively that even though we all find tobacco smoke horrible to begin with, we still hope and expect to come to appreciate it in some way later because we have already been generally convinced that there must be a pleasure somewhere to be had, we just need to persist. Coupled with this is a more basic supposition that there must be *something* in it, or else why would all these other people do it? Obviously smoking must have a *point*. I mean to say: why would millions of people continue doing something that was damaging – for years on end – if it were utterly meaningless and pointless?

To which there is a simple answer: Nail-biting. Compulsive habits can be – and often are – repeated indefinitely without any reason or point to it at all. Look at people who hoard newspapers – or indeed, collect anything. In the case of tobacco we can also add the word 'fashion', which explains all manner of quite unnecessary silliness. (Interestingly enough, fashion is also a form of hypnosis and many people respond to those suggestions without question. In fact very few people are completely immune, because even though lots of us are not very interested in fashion, few people would be happy to be generally regarded as actually 'unfashionable'.)

So when the tobacco companies claimed - during the political debate about the proposed ban on advertising - that they were not trying to encourage non-smokers to start smoking but just attempting to persuade existing smokers to switch brand, they were not being candid. This is obvious since 120,000 smokers die every year from smoking and a whole lot more of them die from other things too. So a promotional policy that only targeted existing smokers – discretion which cannot be ensured anyway in practice, with campaigns aimed at the general public – would be subject to the law of diminishing returns, in a way that makes corporate failure inevitable in due course. No company would deliberately pursue such a course, it would be corporate suicide.

No, they were continuing to add to the mountains of suggestion that had gone before, attempting to perpetuate the notion that smokers enjoy their cigarettes, and suggesting they are just another product you can buy from a shop, like anything else. Another lifestyle choice, associated with leisure and social success. And if you really want to look successful, try these cigars! They were brainwashing all of us, including children and adolescents, fully intending that they would *later* form the notion that the reason they continue to smoke is because they like it, even though they will easily remember that their first smoking experience was revolting.

## Question:

If there is a pleasure in smoking, why didn't we notice it straight away? Was it difficult to spot, or something?

Once we reach this key point about pleasure, during a hypnotherapy session, I will ask the client to focus on the 'pleasure' of smoking, and then describe it to me. Faced with that question, many smokers will recognise all of a sudden that there isn't a pleasure to be found. Light dawns! But not all smokers realise that, by any means. Some are still convinced that there must be a pleasure there somewhere and just assume that I'm wrong to suggest otherwise. Further, they may have an uncomfortable feeling that someone is trying to take that 'pleasure' away, so they dig their heels in and scratch around for something to describe which might pass for 'enjoyment', or an experience worth repeating. And so we hear things like this:

"It's that feeling when the smoke hits the back of your throat..."

"It just gives you that slight buzz, doesn't it?"

"It's really nice to have one after a meal."

"It's the first drag or two, really... not so much the rest of it."

"It's just that feeling of the smoke going down..."

Not very convincing, is it? Given that this behaviour leads to some of the most horrible suffering and hideous deaths that people ever experience, you'd think those people would expect to get a bit more out of it than that, wouldn't you?

The very first time that tobacco smoke hit the back of your throat, you probably nearly threw up. That's how nice it was. That certainly qualifies as a *sensation,* but is it a pleasure? Does it make you feel good? Are we to believe that people spend vast amounts of money over the years, and risk cancer, strokes and heart attacks just for *that*?

Our first experience of the effects of the poison nicotine was that it made us all feel dizzy and sick. To call that a "buzz" is stretching that colloquialism considerably. The feeling of hot, toxic gases filling the airways ("the smoke going down"), however accustomed to it we later become, could never honestly be regarded as a pleasure. And a smoker is not actually *describing* a pleasure if they simply point out *when* it seems satisfying, such as after a meal - that is a fall-back position when you can't answer the actual question. But it does give us a clue as to what is really going on.

Whatever the smoker actually says in answer to the question, I guarantee it will not be a description of pleasure. Some will pause for a while, and then frankly admit they cannot locate any pleasure to describe. Others will search around, sure it must be there somewhere - perhaps describing *when* they do it, or *where* they do it, or *which* cigarettes they like, or don't like during the course of the day. Then when they have finished rambling, I simply ask the original question again, because they did not answer it: "Can you describe the 'pleasure' of inhaling tobacco smoke?"

Many smokers will isolate the first couple of puffs of the cigarette as the bit that seems gratifying, often describing that as a "relief". But if tobacco smoke relieves tension and stress in the smoker, why is it only the first couple of puffs? Surely it should be doing that more and more as you continue smoking the rest of it. "Isn't it really true to say," I point out at this juncture, "that all that actually happens is that the craving goes away as soon as you start smoking, and the 'relief' is just the disappearance of that particular irritation? The stresses and strains of everyday life are still there, they haven't changed in any way – but at least that irritating urge has gone!" It is also apparent that this happens immediately – it is not necessary to smoke the cigarette to bring about that relief by degrees, as would be the case if the relief were truly a result of ingesting the nicotine content of the whole cigarette. This confirms that the urge is to *light* a cigarette, not to smoke it – and indeed many smokers put them out without smoking the whole thing, or leave them burning in an ashtray and forget all about them, or even light up another.

Now add the simple fact that the smoker may well be relaxing or taking a break at that moment, which is a lot more pleasant than not being on a break. This additional relaxation factor is real of course, but it isn't coming from the smoke – yet tobacco often gets the credit for that too, in the smoker's mind.

## The First Shock: It's Horrible!

By the time we actually try it for ourselves, usually in teenage years, tobacco is already filed away in the mind under 'Pleasures' because of the advertising and our collective associated assumptions. 'Adult Pleasures', to be exact. What are we interested in during the teenage years? Turning ourselves from children into adults, and getting our hands on adult stuff. So all this comes up on the agenda.

Now, we do get a bit of a shock when we first try tobacco. Not only is there a conspicuous lack of pleasure, it turns out to be absolutely bloody horrible and it nearly knocks us over. But as teenagers, we assume that this is because tobacco is really for grown-ups. Presumably, the reason we find it pretty hard to take is because we are little more than kids, and shouldn't be doing it anyway. This is not something we are likely to admit in front of our friends: "You know, I don't think I'm old enough to like this yet!" No, because the whole point of doing it is to look more grown up and less like a kid. So we mask our disgust and nausea as best we can, and try to look as if we are actually enjoying the inhalation of poisonous fumes. Most of all we try not to heave, because that would not be cool.

When I was a youngster, and adopting the smoking pose for the first time I knew I found it a revolting experience, but I was always under the impression that my friends actually did like smoking tobacco, because they acted as if they did. But then, so did I! It was only many years later when I got into discussing this with hundreds of adult smokers, that I realised the truth. None of us enjoyed inhaling cigarette fumes, we all found it most unpleasant really. We might have pretended that we enjoyed smoking, but in reality, it was exactly like the Emperor's New Clothes: nobody objected because nobody wanted to look stupid. But if just one brave leader had had the wit to say: "Look, this is absolutely horrible isn't it? What the hell are we doing this for?" ...then we could all have dropped it right then and there, and moved right along to sampling beer and actually enjoying ourselves for real.

However, no such wondrous thing occurred. So we all carried on puffing away, mainly just because we weren't supposed to be doing it. We were rebels! Personally, I was also hoping it made me look tougher, but it probably didn't. When I look at thirteen-year-old kids smoking now, I realise what I must have looked like: awkward, self-conscious, queasy and utterly thirteen.

Later on, we just became accustomed to the nausea and stopped noticing it most of the time. Of course you notice it all over again when you are ill, or have a hangover. Or if you haven't had a cigarette for quite a while, then the nausea might become noticeable again briefly. Or if you try smoking a cigarette that is very different from the brand you are accustomed to smoking. That is when you hear yourself saying to the provider: "How can you smoke these? They're horrible!"

Actually they are all horrible. You are just not accustomed to those.

It never becomes nice. What actually happens is that later on, smoking becomes attached to certain particular moments in the day, some of which are pleasant *moments,* for some other reason. When I ask clients if they enjoy smoking, the most common answer I get is "Sometimes." So I ask when those times are, and they immediately point to these particular moments in the day:

"First thing in the morning, when I sit down with my cup of tea before I really get going..."

"Break from work..."

"After a meal..."

"Out for a drink with friends – that's when I really enjoy a cigarette!"

Actually, that's when you are really *enjoying yourself* – you just happen to be smoking at the same time. The pleasure there is real, it is just not coming from the cigarette, because if cigarettes could 'cause pleasure' then they all would, they are all exactly the same - including the first one you tried, which knocked you sick. "In fact," I tell the client, "the good news is that you are not giving up a pleasure at all, because it has been masquerading as a pleasure all along. It is really just breathing smoke in and out – how nice could it possibly be, under any circumstances?

## The Evidence for 'Pleasure' is Entirely Circumstantial

Smokers often comment that they no longer smoke at work at all, because nowadays they would have to go down four flights of stairs, walk 150 yards to a silly little 'shelter' and stand there only partially protected from the wind and rain, self-consciously puffing miserably away on a coffin-nail, in full view of everyone in the area. This 'provision' for the needs of smokers could hardly be less comfortable. It might still just about qualify as a break, but this relief is countered by inconvenience, lack of comfortable furniture, exposure to the elements and (let's face it) shame. This is not enjoyable.

## Back in the Good Old Days...

Before smoking in enclosed public places was banned in the UK, it was much easier to believe that smoking itself was pleasurable. Take the example of smoking in public houses for example: when smokers were in the pub, of course they were enjoying themselves. They were not working, for one thing. They were enjoying the leisure time, the relaxation, the atmosphere, the company, the conversation, the alcohol – all these can generate good feelings. Inhaling tobacco smoke doesn't, we noticed that on Day One. But later on we had forgotten that, and in the pub situation, tobacco was just lumped in there with everything else, we don't notice the difference.

In truth, tobacco smoke is the one element that can be taken out of that scenario without pleasure being reduced one iota, because it wasn't contributing any – *provided* the craving is taken out too, which is where hypnotherapy comes in. Because if any pre-ban smoker tried to quit just with willpower and then went to the pub, cravings would drive them up the wall. And then it would seem for all the world as if the only reason they were able to enjoy relaxing in the pub is because they were still inhaling the fumes from burning dead leaves, when the truth was that their Subconscious mind was using the craving system to prompt the usual smoking behaviour in the usual situations, quite unaware of the conscious decision to quit. In that pre-ban scenario, other smokers would still be lighting up, so it was evidently okay to do so. Others lighting up would also have prompted more craving signals, as it functions as a suggestion.

This is exactly why many smokers opposed the ban on smoking in pubs. They feared they would not be able to relax or enjoy themselves in the pub without tobacco. They needn't have worried, on two counts: smoking 'shelters' have been built at the back of many pubs anyway for the die-hard smokers, and in any case most smokers will simply adjust their habit subconsciously according to the new reality. Just like on buses, in cinemas, on aircraft and so on. Once the brain catches on that this particular space is no longer a smoking opportunity – because nobody is doing it now - it stops sending the signal whilst the smoker is in that space. The vast majority of smokers will have noticed that fact already. Sadly for the people who ran ordinary pubs, quite a lot of smokers quit the pub anyway at that point, either because of the fear or just to rebel against the new restriction, or perhaps a bit of both. So the traditional role of the public house – the place working men went to after work, to drink away their wages before eventually arriving home pissed, throwing their dinner at the wall and terrifying their wife and children... was dealt yet another tragic blow.

## Smoking Gestures: Real Aims and Body Language

After the initial shock of discovering how horrible tobacco smoke is, there is a fairly rapid adjustment. If we subsequently came to believe that smoking was indeed pleasurable, what changed was *our perception of it* – the smoke itself didn't change a bit. Were we wrong, back then? Did we get the wrong end of the stick at first, fail to see the beauty of it, miss the joy to be had? Not at all. Pleasure is either there in the actual experience or it is not. If it had been, we would have noticed that straight away. The truth is, we had *other reasons* for choosing to smoke cigarettes. The attraction was never in the physical experience - which was sickening - but in *acting out the smoking behaviour,* which was

reckoned to be 'cool'. It is initially a performance, a statement, which can be signalling a number of different things:
1. An act of rebellion, defying authority.
2. A statement of independence, or a coming of age.
3. "Mirroring" or copying behaviour within a social group.
4. Adopting a style or an attitude, usually based on an iconic figure.

The mirroring factor is described by Allan Pease in *Body Language:*

> This 'carbon copying' is a means by which one person tells the other that he is in agreement with his ideas and attitudes. By this method, one is non-verbally saying to the other, "As you can see, I think the same as you, so I will copy your posture and gestures".

This is highly significant because smoking always begins as a response to suggestion. If the dominant figures within any group smoke, then smoking behaviour is endorsed generally and others are likely to follow. Allan Pease again:

> Research shows that when the leader of a group uses certain gestures and positions, subordinates copy them.

Smoking behaviour incorporates many gestures, and signals many attitudes. Long before we smoke ourselves, we learn them all: from film and photographic imagery featuring movie stars like James Dean and Humphrey Bogart, from popular musicians, from tobacco advertising (e.g. the Marlboro Man) as well as from family and friends. These are old references now, but they were very influential in their time. Later, when such overt promotion became discouraged, it allowed up-and-coming, 'edgy' new stars to appear rebellious by allowing themselves to be photographed smoking anyway, and the rise of cannabis use too became 'endorsed' by iconic images of people like Bob Marley. The fact that Marley died from lung cancer in his thirties somehow doesn't seem to make images of him with a joint in his mouth any less cool, at least for his many admirers.

Some people choose to be, or end up being loners (the James Dean type), and may adopt a particular smoking attitude without joining a group. Their style of smoking may signal a rejection of others: "I don't need you, I've got my cigarettes" - a slightly different take on "You're never alone with a Strand". Notice also how many of this type will roll their own cigarettes – again, a statement of difference and independence, a rejection even of other smokers. The all-important *sharing* gestures, usually common amongst young smokers are then made awkward, deliberately. And whilst the endless fiddling with papers and dried leaves is going on, the world can be pointedly ignored by the loner. (Of course, to have its full effect, this must be *seen by others* – you can't play the loner in society effectively if you are genuinely absent. James Dean epitomises this: he played the loner before thousands of adoring, mesmerized movie fans, who were ironically 'with him' all the way.)

Some people choose to be leaders, and if they decide to adopt smoking gestures as part of their act, they will probably be modelling themselves on some leader that has gone before. Their smoking behaviour will say a lot about their style of leadership: forceful and 'in your face', or thoughtful, moody and obscured behind a cloud of smoke (difficult to read). There are various ways to use smoke if you are a leader, it can be both a weapon and a shield. It can also be a bonding ritual, symbolising acceptance or allegiance like the Native American peace pipe ritual, or the modern equivalent of handing out expensive cigars. In the U.K., tobacco taxes are so high nowadays that even handing round a packet of cigarettes in company can seem pretty generous.

If neither a loner nor a leader, the rest will tend to be followers of one sort or another. Their smoking is inspired mainly by the leaders in the group, and they will be influenced by the style of smoking the leaders adopt. It becomes a group attitude, along with many other facets of the group's identity. Soon it all becomes habit and the influence of others will diminish, but it never quite disappears. In nearly all cases of relapse, someone else present was smoking at the moment of relapse. We all like to think that we just do as we please, of course, but hardly anyone is so socially inept as to be unaware of body language, and how to react with familiar social gestures. "Smoking, eh? I'll join you!" has a more convivial air than "Do you *have* to smoke in here? Since I stopped I can't bear the smell I'm afraid. No offence."

On the other hand, "Throat biopsy, eh? I'll join you!" does not seem quite so jolly, does it? Really it is just breathing toxic gases in and out, how pleasant could it possibly be on any occasion?

One lady actually said to me, with a straight face: "It's my only pleasure in life." I said: "You might as well shoot yourself, then." I think she was a bit shocked. But not quite shocked enough, so I added: "If inhaling poisonous gases from burning dead leaves was really the only aspect of your existence you could regard as pleasant, you would be better off dead. In fact I would load the gun for you myself if I thought that were really true. It would be the kindest thing to do – to put you out of your misery." She didn't look as if she thought that would be kind at all – clients don't expect their therapist to encourage them to commit suicide - but I was using the shock tactic to get the message home. Of course it wasn't true: lots of things in life are more pleasant than inhaling fumes. She was just taking all those things for granted and repeating something she had heard other smokers say many times but without really thinking about it.

Smokers often repeat suggestions other smokers have said before, in order to try to maintain the illusion of conscious choice in their own minds. The more often a suggestion is repeated, the more plausible it sounds: "Why quit," smokers often ask one another, "when you could get knocked down by a bus tomorrow?" Not very likely to happen though, is it? Buses are huge, you can see them coming a mile off. They usually don't move very fast, they make lots of noise and they are often painted yellow or red. You would have to be incredibly careless to actually get knocked down by a bus.

Lung cancer sneaks up on people. By the time you know you've got that, you are in deep trouble already. Mouth cancer, heart attacks, strokes, blood clots - these things suddenly hit the smoker out of a clear blue sky, and all the plausible devil-may-care bullshit in the world won't help you then. Whether you regard tobacco smoking as a pleasure or not, it's not worth dying for, is it? No pleasure is worth dying for, even if it is bloody fantastic. And let's face it, the old coffin nails were never that. Ask any thirteen-year-old.

### b). "I'm hooked, I am addicted, that's why I do it."

Lots of smokers believe they are addicted, and I believe I have already destroyed that argument in Section Five, Volume I.

### c). "It is very hard to stop smoking, everybody says so."

It is not surprising smokers tend to believe it is very hard to stop smoking because the methods they are using do not work for most people. They are simply the wrong methods. I would agree that it is very difficult to succeed with those methods, but with hypnotherapy it is effortless. Before people ever try hypnotherapy though, they usually try various other methods which have very low success rates. It is rare for any smoker to try hypnotherapy first.

The first method of choice for the would-be quitter is likely to be willpower. This is unlikely to succeed permanently, for reasons I explain in Section 12. The next thing they try is usually the thing that is plastered all over every pharmacy shop-front: nicotine, the poison that became a medicine. Ooh, I've just realised that sounds like a lovely story, doesn't it? "The Poison that Became a Medicine", what a heart-warming bedtime tale! A bit like The Selfish Giant. Anyway that doesn't work either, although the poor smoker might try all the various vehicles the poison goes about in, before they come to that sad conclusion. They start with the gum, then try the patches, the lozenges, the microtab and finally the one they can have fun loading and fiddling about with: the pen/pipe/dummy "inhalator" device with the nicotine cartridge. I'm surprised it's not also a camera.

In fact, "Collect them all!" Then once you've got the set and find you are still miserably puffing away on the old cancer sticks, you realise it is time for drastic action. It's off to the GP to see if you can try that Wonder Drug you read about in the newspaper: bupropion, or "Zyban" as it is more memorably known. This has a better success rate than all those nicotine things, possibly as high as 25% according to some sources, although others reckon 13% at best. Amongst the unfortunate side effects, though, is the possibility of severe personality changes resulting in depression and maybe even suicide - but don't let that put you off. It still counts as stopping smoking. And to be fair, most people who try Zyban do not commit suicide as a result. Most of them don't stop smoking permanently either. Although it is undeniable that the *most* permanent smoking cessation cases achieved by Zyban are inevitably within that small group who killed themselves after taking it. There is no doubt that they will never smoke again, so draw what conclusions you will from those facts. Did they kill themselves because of Zyban? Well we can never know for sure, but what we do know for sure is that various other methods are 100% safe and more successful too, so:

## On to Other Methods!

Some smokers then get all alternative, and try acupuncture or some herbal remedy. Various alternative therapies offer help with stopping smoking, or other habits/addictions. And indeed they may help: it is clear that acupuncture scored higher than NRT in the study by the University of Iowa detailed in Section Nine, Volume I. Also, that study may not show these alternative options at their best. The hypnotherapy methods studied were so basic and flawed that it makes us wonder what level of expertise was involved in the acupuncture that was also being assessed. Anyone can stick a nicotine patch on, but hypnotherapy and acupuncture require expert knowledge, skill, experience and talent if you want to see the best results possible with those methods.

It is not uncommon for smokers to come to hypnotherapy last, after having tried all those other things, by which point they are pretty much convinced that it is very hard to stop smoking and that they are unable to do it. They are also expecting very little help from any method at this point. Then the hypnotherapist starts telling them it is *easy?* How ready are they to believe that, after all that struggle and disappointment? "You are my last hope!" is a forlorn statement hypnotherapists hear often.

The fact is, hypnotherapy is by far the most successful method of permanently eliminating the smoking habit when it is conducted effectively, because it is the only method that treats the problem for what it really is - a compulsive habit. NRT is Not Really Therapy because it is barking up the wrong tree in the first place. The different types of NRT really just equate to barking up the wrong tree wearing different collars.

Zyban is notoriously unpredictable and certainly involves some risk, whereas acupuncture is not risky at all and you are more likely to succeed with it anyway. Hypnotherapy is the best, the safest, usually the quickest and certainly the easiest option for the majority. No wonder people tend to assume it sounds too good to be true if they have little or no personal experience of it, because they are so accustomed to the idea that it is difficult to stop smoking, or indeed change any other habit.

Then we have the latest anti-smoking pill to arrive, Champix, made by Pfizer. This became available in the UK on prescription in July 2007, a twice-daily tablet course over 12 weeks, costing the NHS £163 per patient. This was reported to have a "success rate" of 44% in trials, beating another drug which managed 30% and a placebo which scored 18%. But that 44% figure was NOT the real success rate, it was the percentage not smoking at the end of the 12 week trial. Anyone who read Volume I will know already that this sort of statistic usually bears no relation to the results at one year, as we saw with Nicotine Replacement Poisoning. The Department of Health claimed an average national quit rate of 53% for that in one press release, which as we know dwindled to a miserable 6% at one year. It was always highly likely that we were going to see that happen all over again. Even in the original drug trials, a follow-up study showed that half of that 44% were smoking again 28 weeks later.

## Oh No! Not the Nicotine Tale Again

It is claimed that Champix works by blocking the 'nicotine receptors' in the brain, thus reducing 'the need for nicotine'. Since craving signals are not caused by a 'need for nicotine' anyway, the entire principle is based on a myth. It has also been claimed that the drug 'reduces the pleasure' of smoking. This would be difficult to achieve since there is no real pleasure in smoking anyway, only the illusion of it. Certainly Champix causes nausea in a lot of people, perhaps enough to put them off smoking for long enough for the habit to be broken. The trouble with that is, the drug is only supposed to be prescribed for twelve weeks, you can't stay on it. Since none of the ideas and beliefs supporting the smoking habit have even been addressed - and certainly not at a Subconscious level - what do you suppose will happen next time there is a stag do, a girls' night out, a Christmas party, somebody's $21^{st}$, a wedding or a trip to Amsterdam?

Oh, and there is just one other small problem with Champix. Quite a number of smokers have killed themselves whilst taking it, many of them having never had any previous history of mental illness. And it has caused a disturbing number of other serious reactions too, some of which don't seem to go away even when the smoker stops taking Champix. The horror story is still unfolding as this book goes into production.

## New drug to stop whistling and nail-biting: coming soon!

None of this dangerous medication is necessary. Habitual behaviour is not set in stone: the Subconscious can change it any time you like, and on request. As Allen Carr rightly pointed out, here in the UK we are in the habit of driving on the left, yet if we drive on the continent we break that habit without any real difficulty at all. What he failed to appreciate is that we effectively have no choice in his example, whereas with smoking there usually is a choice, so he is wrong to imply that stopping smoking should be just as easy, simply a logical step. But it does demonstrate that habits are not really outside your control at all, merely outside your *conscious* control. Your Subconscious is controlling it fine, and would normally have no idea you made a conscious decision to change it.

In the driving example, the Subconscious really has no other option than to adjust to the unfamiliar reality. With smoking, it usually does that anyway in places where smoking is not an option. But when it comes to a new conscious decision to eliminate the habit completely, hypnotherapy is the only way to explain the new decision and the reasons for it to the Subconscious, in detail, and in a language to which the Subconscious can easily relate. This procedure is not difficult at all for the client, who does not even have to be paying attention on a conscious level for it to be perfectly successful, and doesn't have to believe in hypnotherapy either until the results prove their conscious expectations to be wrong about that. It doesn't even matter if they have some mixed feelings about quitting – that's normal, and we take care of that during the session. They only need to have a genuine preference to be rid of the problem, and a positive attitude to that change.

## The Conscious Mind Does Not Expect Success

It is normal for the conscious mind to be astonished by the success of hypnotherapy. However positive the new client is trying to be, their conscious mind expects failure, or half-expects it. That is why clients typically react with delight and astonishment when they get exciting results. They say things like: "It's incredible!" and "It's astonishing, I can't believe it, everyone is amazed!" They would not be talking like that if those results were exactly what everyone had expected.

This is not simply because people cannot help being negative, although that is also the case with some clients. It is because the conscious mind is trained to be logical. So when it is trying to guess what the future holds, it has to base that guess on hard evidence, not what some therapist claims the outcome should be. The only hard evidence the client has is their previous experience of attempts to stop smoking, so the client's conscious mind is forever looking *back* to guess what the future probably holds: "So we're here to stop smoking. Let's see: stopping smoking... that usually means *struggle* and *failure,* let's project that into the future as our likely conscious expectation."

In doing this, the conscious mind is not trying to be negative. It is trying to be accurate based on the story so far. But this does not prevent a successful outcome, because their Subconscious mind neither knows nor cares what the conscious mind thinks or expects. The Subconscious mind will do what it likes, and when that turns out to be positive change, the conscious mind will always be pleasantly surprised because it wasn't really expecting that. This is part of the fun of doing hypnotherapy.

However, this factor can also function as the one major drawback of hypnotherapy in private practice, because if the Subconscious holds back on positive change at first, for some reason, the conscious mind might immediately assume it was 'right all along about this hypnotherapy nonsense', and can get quite stroppy, as if the therapist has pulled a fast one and swindled them out of their money.

In reality it is quite rare for people to take that attitude, but it does happen sometimes and hypnotherapists occasionally have to square up to a client who has suddenly adopted a hostile attitude, stand their ground and explain why the client is not due a refund - just as they are not due a refund from the pharmacist when the patches don't work. You buy in therapy at your own risk, obviously, not at the risk of the provider. Most people understand that anyway, and just come back for further therapy, which usually pays off anyway. For the therapist, a philosophical attitude to outcomes develops over time. You can't win 'em all, but we do win so many that the few negative outcomes actually become essential, just so we can still get our heads through doorways. Frequent success can make any one of us cocky or complacent, so ironically, whilst the occasional disappointing outcome is certainly not good for that client, it can be therapeutic for the therapist, who is reminded that they are not a miracle-worker despite what their more successful clients may tell them.

The client's success is the *client's* success... as are all outcomes in reality.

I'll deal with the next two together, as they are almost the same idea:

### d). & e). "It relaxes me," and "It helps me deal with stress."

No, it doesn't: smoking makes your heart beat faster and your blood pressure rise. That is not relaxing and actually causes physical stress within the cardio-vascular system. This can prove fatal especially if you are over thirty years of age. But if you are fairly young and fit, you wouldn't notice your heart beating faster. You certainly don't know what your blood pressure is even if it is dangerously high, so those particular effects of nicotine are usually not noticed by smokers at all. They certainly aren't *aiming* to increase heart-rate or blood pressure.

So how did any of us get the impression that smoking was relaxing us, if it was actually doing the reverse? Originally from tobacco advertising, just like the notion of pleasure. We grew up surrounded by thousands of images of people 'relaxing' with a Benson & Hedges, or a cigar. For many years, we couldn't pick up a magazine without noticing that the back page featured a photograph of some chap lazing in an easy chair with a brandy glass in one hand and a burning cigarette in the other. The visual suggestion comprises: comfy, lazy, contented, happy, relaxing, brandy & smoke. The brand-name of the tobacco product is attached to the appealing image, as if the *smoke* produced the relaxing feelings that are implied by the image.

In truth, those feelings would really be produced by a combination of factors: brandy, an easy chair, being comfortably positioned and having nothing demanding to do at that moment. The advertisers are trying to persuade you that the smoke – and specifically this brand – should actually get the credit for that. "You want to feel as comfortable as this guy? Then buy a pack of these!" That is the suggestion, and it is dishonest, because you certainly won't feel like that unless you include all the other factors too. In truth, the tobacco is the one thing you can leave out of the picture without reducing your relaxation at all, because it wasn't contributing any.

So the idea of 'relaxation' was drilled into all of us, just like the 'pleasure' suggestion, long before we ever smoked ourselves. When we first tried smoking in teenage years, none of our smoking friends said to us: "Try one of these, it will really relax you!" No-one suggested it would help us deal with stress either. It's not that you don't have any stress as a teenager – I seem to remember those years being very stressful, in fact – it's just that smoking was never about that in the first place. We had other reasons, at the time, for learning how to strike a suitable smoking pose. Those relaxation notions come back into play later, when the teenage stuff is all history and you realise that you apparently cannot stop smoking. Now you regard it as a problem, and you need something to tell yourself about why you are doing this. When we are thirteen we know exactly what we find exciting about sneaking off somewhere with a packet of cigarettes, and it has nothing to do with the effects of the smoke, which we just find sickening.

Once the suggestion of relaxation has been established in the mind of the smoker – which it was long before smoking actually started – later on four factors seem to confirm and reinforce the idea:

1. The fact that other people often repeat the relaxation suggestion, either verbally or via their body language (lighting up with a sigh and stretching out).
2. The fact that smokers tend to smoke at moments of repose, not when they are busy, when it would just get in the way. So smoking episodes often *coincide* with relaxing moments, such as taking a break, sitting down with a drink, going out and socialising etc.
3. The fact that cravings are themselves annoying, so if the Subconscious reacts to a tense or demanding situation by triggering a craving – as a direct result of all the millions of advertising suggestions that smoking will relax you - that craving winds you up even further. The moment you light up, it disappears immediately, which is of course a relief. This is not truly a relief from the stress of the demanding situation, except that you might now also be taking a break from the situation. If you have successfully got away from the source of the irritation, then the solution can be misread by the smoker, and the cigarette might get the credit for what the break actually achieved. Otherwise the only relief is the disappearance of the added irritation of the craving, so your net result in terms of stress relief from the cigarette itself is nil.
4. The fact that we originally learned what smoking was *apparently* for by watching other people do it. We

regularly saw smokers lighting up with a sigh, and stretching out, all through our childhood - which does create the suggestion that the cigarette makes you feel like that. In reality, the gestures of physical relaxation are coinciding with *lighting up,* not smoking the cigarette. It is *instant* relaxation. No drug works that fast even if you inject it. The smoker simply intends and expects to relax at that moment, so they do. Tension and relaxation are muscular states, real bodily experiences defined by our emotional response to a situation. 'Lighting up' = 'Time to relax' so the smoker does exactly that. Also this coincides with the irritation of the craving disappearing, so it seems to confirm the suggestion that something in the smoke is relaxing them. In fact the smokers are doing the 'relaxing' themselves, it isn't coming from the smoke. What *is* coming from the smoke will shortly afterwards make their heart beat faster and their blood pressure rise, but they probably will not notice that... unless of course they have a heart attack.

As I pointed out in Section Ten (Volume I), when I compared tobacco smoking with nail-biting, what people do when they are under stress is one thing. Whether it is genuinely useful is another. The conscious mind of the smoker may try to claim that smoking brings relief from stress because it has long been aware of that notion, and it also observes that the reaction to stress and conflict appears to be an urge to reach for a cigarette. So it mistakes the prompt for a bodily need, assumes that need is real and that the cigarette or the nicotine will fulfil that need. Yet the same smoker can clearly see that the nail-biter's reaction to stress is destructive and useless, and only makes them appear tense and anxious. When they learn that nicotine increases their blood pressure and their heart-rate too, they are confused because they have never noticed that. They have noticed, though, that the irritating signal prompting the smoker to light up goes away when they light up, which is a relief in itself.

So the smoker clearly sees the nail-biter's response as an anxiety reaction which doesn't really help, but fails to recognise that the same is true of their own response. The smoker has a similar reaction – when the stress levels go up, they smoke more – but the smoker might be under the impression that they are doing that on purpose because it helps - a potentially lethal notion resulting in many individual deaths every day. This is why so many smokers suffer heart attacks and strokes because they do not know what nicotine does anyway, and they reach for the cigarettes at the worst moment they could possibly pick. It overloads the system and down they go with a heart attack.

Now this isn't likely to happen when you are twenty, because the system is strong and can withstand the extra pressure. But as we get older, the internal plumbing develops the odd weak spot here and there, which we don't know anything about because they are all on the inside – and which might not cause a problem ordinarily, but stress puts that weak point under more physical strain. If you then add nicotine on top of that it can suddenly become a fatal combination even though it wasn't quite so deadly when you were younger and fitter. The fact that smoking rarely proves fatal during the first years of doing it lulls the smoker into a false sense of security. There are often very nasty surprises further down the line, but because the conscious mind generally expects today to be roughly similar to yesterday, it doesn't expect today's pack of cigarettes to trigger a heart attack precisely because none of the thousands of previous packs did. And it will go on assuming that right up until the enormous shock of the first heart attack.

### f). "It helps me concentrate at work."

Who can smoke at work these days? Well a few people still are allowed to, usually because they work for themselves, or another smoker. I could smoke at work myself, I suppose – although I'd rather lose a finger than become a smoker again. Years ago when

I was a university lecturer I often noticed that when I was marking coursework or exam papers I seemed to smoke excessively. Since I was usually a 'light' smoker, I wondered about this and I can understand why some smokers assume that smoking helps them to concentrate.

I also noticed however – and quite a few colleagues confessed to me that they observed the same thing in themselves, as did students – that when I had marking or writing to do I would get repeated cravings for food and drink as well. I was forever in the fridge looking for snacks even though I wasn't really hungry, or making myself cups of tea I wouldn't normally be bothering with.

Now that I am a hypnotherapist I can explain it and indeed cure it. This often comes up as a feature of sessions we do on concentration, or study and revision for exams. The key factor here is that there is no *desire* to do this sort of work. We might resolve to do it, and we might have all sorts of good reasons for aiming to succeed with it, but these are all conscious aims and intentions. Deep down inside most of us would actually prefer to do something easier or more entertaining, like read a book, watch TV or go to the pub. We are forcing ourselves to mark these exam papers, either because our professional position obliges us to do that, or just for money. These are two matters the Subconscious mind knows nothing about. The only thing the Subconscious knows is that we don't really want to do this, do we? This is boring, tiring and miserable – why are we doing this? So it keeps offering an 'out' using the craving system. It keeps sending little nudges with a feeling attached suggesting one thing or another 'might be nice'. The conscious mind instantly follows that up with a rationalisation, which I have underlined in each case:

*Nudge!* A nice cool drink, that's what we could do with! <u>Then we can get on with it, thinks the conscious mind</u>. So we get a nice cool drink, and settle down to do some more, but there's the nudge again:

*Nudge!* What about a packet of crisps? Oh, okay – back to the kitchen – no crisps, but I could make a sandwich, so spend five minutes doing that... then we can really get some work done. Settle down again, but actually I'm not working now, I'm eating a sandwich. So might as well finish eating that before we can really get started again... there. Now then... where was I?

*Nudge!* Let's have a cigarette and really get down to it... where's my cigarettes? Did I leave them in the kitchen? Back to the kitchen... but by the time I get there (*Nudge!*) I've forgotten the cigarettes because I've just 'remembered'...

...that strawberry flan in the fridge. Because that needs eating... so I arrive back at the stack of unmarked exam papers with strawberry flan. I'll get going in a minute, I really will. But after the strawberry flan (*Nudge!*) of course I 'remember':

The cigarettes. And when I do locate them, I find there are only two left (*accessing & supplies nudge*) – what time is it? I'd better get to the shop now, or I'll end up having to drive to the all-night garage, and that will only waste more time I could otherwise spend marking. At the shop I bump into a colleague who is just off to the pub... and since it is now a straight spontaneous choice between the marking I wasn't really doing anyway and a golden opportunity to sack it in favour of a pint, the Subconscious has no hesitation in administering the coup de grace to that particular attempt to get some work done: *Go on, have a lovely pint – you can do that other shit later!*

...and so the next morning finds us with a stack of unmarked papers and a hangover. How did that happen? Again.

What this demonstrates is that the Subconscious mind is very good at thwarting conscious intentions it knows nothing about just by giving us "better ideas" via the craving system. On a Subconscious level there is no desire whatever to do the work – that's why it is called "work" – and the urge to light up is only one of many opportunities it is offering us to *do something else,* it is just that the conscious mind doesn't realise this. It also explains why there is such a strong mental connection between smoking and 'taking a break' from work. These are breaks the non-smoker feels no urge to take anyway, although the non-smoker may get similar urges to visit the vending machine or the coffee-maker. Of course, for the poor unfortunate who can still smoke at their desk – like those who work at home, for example – this usually develops into a habit of smoking heavily while working, and so then there is no break unless it is going to be a trip to the fridge or the drinks machine. This person will almost certainly believe they are smoking more to 'help them concentrate' but actually they have to keep lighting up repeatedly to get rid of the distractions the Subconscious was deliberately throwing in, so that they can then continue to concentrate normally.

It is very easy to get these distractions removed in therapy. We simply explain to the Subconscious the information it does not possess: that there are good reasons for getting the work done, and avoiding it has consequences the Subconscious wasn't taking into account because it knew nothing of them. Career responsibilities, or advancement and financial considerations are all matters taken care of by the conscious mind. Once it is explained in detail and repeated a few times just to get it properly established, the Subconscious will happily remove these distractions from then on. It was only trying to help, but was unaware of the conscious resolve or the reasons behind it. The Subconscious was simply judging by your lack of *desire* to undertake those tasks, and directing effective avoidance strategies. It is quite happy to stop, if those signals were inappropriate for some reason it knew nothing about.

### g). "It helps me keep my weight down."

For many people - especially women - this is the number one 'reason' for delaying any attempt to quit. If this is a concern of yours, please read this section very carefully, maybe a few times – because there is no need to be afraid of this factor, weight-gain is easily prevented by expert hypnotherapy.

If smoking genuinely helped people keep their weight down, there would be no fat smokers. But in any case, as methods of weight control go, smoking is far more damaging than anorexia or bulimia, because it kills more people than both of those conditions put together. Just consider this shocking fact:

> The UK suffers thousands of deaths every year through road accidents, accidents at home and at work, murder and manslaughter, suicide, poisoning, overdoses and HIV infection. Smoking kills around six times more people than *all these put together*.
>
> *from:* Don't Stop Smoking Until You've Read This Book, Adler&Morris, HowToBooks 2002

As an attempt to control weight, smoking is potentially suicidal, certainly unhealthy, costly and pretty unreliable anyway. It is true that stopping smoking can trigger weight gain in some people, but here's the good news: effective hypnotherapy can prevent it entirely by eliminating the four causes. How long does this take? No more than about five minutes. We take care of it during the Stop Smoking session. In about 10% of cases a back-up session is required as well, but only because those people did not respond appropriately to the suggestions about weight and food in the first session.

How much does hypnotherapy actually cost? Well, that will vary a bit but it certainly won't cost an arm and a leg. Smoking does: a smoking habit usually ends up costing tens of thousands of pounds, and it is not unheard of for smoking to end up costing a person their legs too, if they don't die of cancer or a heart attack first. And I suppose losing your legs is technically weight loss but it isn't really the kind of weight loss smokers are hoping for when they have a cigarette instead of breakfast.

Weight control is not the subject of this book, but it is the most popular reason for people walking into my office. It is tremendous fun to do that therapy because it is nothing like dieting and people are so amazed and delighted by the results. Results happen quickly for most people and it is easy to sustain the results. You don't need willpower and the great thing is that the weight usually does not go back on afterwards - it stays off, which is different from what usually happens after dieting.

Does that sound too good to be true? Well if it does, that is because you are much more familiar with the dictates of the Dieting Industry as an approach to weight loss, and therefore accustomed to doing things the hard way and getting poor or temporary results. Your conscious mind may already have given up hope, expecting it to always be that way – but if so, your conscious mind is wrong!

When people with a weight issue first hear that hypnotherapy can solve that problem, most of them do not bother to try it anyway, purely because of numerous previous attempts to succeed that did not involve hypnotherapy. This is a bit like the lost soul crawling through the desert parched with thirst, but ignoring the real oasis because: "It's bound to be just another mirage, and I don't want another disappointment like the last one". Diets always promise to solve the problem, and at first you might lose weight temporarily but you always end up back where you started, or even heavier than you were before. So serial dieters steadily lose faith in weight loss programmes - including hypnotherapy which they may never have actually tried. Also, it sounds too easy – even dieting didn't bring long-term success, and that was really difficult, so how can something as effortless as hypnotherapy succeed? This is how the conscious mind talks itself out of new routes for positive change.

# How Hypnotherapy Prevents Weight Gain When Smokers Quit

The four causes of weight gain that hypnotherapy eliminates:

1. Trying to 'Feed' Cravings Away

When people try to stop smoking by any method *except hypnotherapy,* the cravings will still be experienced. All craving signals are similar because they are all 'reminder' signals from the Subconscious. So a signal telling you it is time to smoke a cigarette will feel quite similar to the signal that it is time for a sandwich, or a coffee. Bear in mind that these feelings do not truly indicate a real *need* for anything contained in the sandwich, or the coffee, or the cigarette smoke – it is just a prompt, a nudging reminder that "usually you'd have one of these round about now, wouldn't you?" Expert hypnotherapy shuts down those signals entirely, eliminating that problem.

What should you do if you have hypnotherapy, but are still bothered later by cravings? Simple: consult your therapist, or if you don't have much faith in them, find a more expert therapist. Also, read *How to Choose a Good Hypnotherapist* in Section 15.

2. The Effect of Suggestion Over Many Years

Suggestion has a powerful effect on the way we feel and think, and therefore on the way we behave. It also affects our expectations, all of which conditions our actual experience. Suggestion isn't something we only respond to in trance, we are bombarded by suggestion all the time whether in trance or not, and we are going to respond to some of it sometimes. All advertising, for example, is suggestion – and if it didn't work, of course manufacturers and service providers would not waste millions of pounds doing it. It can work very effectively, especially when the ad people get it right because it deliberately plays upon our *fears* and/or our *desires.* In other words, advertising is usually aimed at the Subconscious mind.

Of course we can all flatter ourselves that we're personally far too intelligent to be influenced by mere suggestion but any human being who really believes that is seriously deluded. Even professional masters of suggestion - like hypnotherapists, advertisers, sales people and their criminal alter-ego, the con-man – none of these people are entirely immune to suggestion themselves, because we all have fears and desires. It doesn't matter how skeptical the conscious, rational mind is about any suggestion it is yet possible for the Subconscious to accept it anyway and overrule the conscious mind entirely.

Two factors decide this:

a. the extent of desire or 'need'
b. the extent of fear.

You will have heard the suggestion that people balloon up in weight or begin to eat compulsively if they stop smoking dozens of times over many years, in many different contexts. Usually it is based upon subjective reports of real individual experience, but only concerning people who have quit smoking the hard way (i.e. without hypnotherapy), and those people will have been unaware how any of these four key factors were affecting them and thereby actually causing the problem. Weight-gain following stopping smoking is not a foregone conclusion because it is not caused by the fact of no longer smoking, but the way the change was handled. Those who gain weight would not have known that these factors are easily removed with hypnosis, and some of these people return to smoking because they are alarmed by the sudden weight increase which is immediately damaging to their self-esteem (and possibly relationships also), so it can take precedence over apparently less-immediate risks to health such as cancer, which the smoker is usually in denial about anyway. Until they actually get cancer, that is.

Now here's how suggestion works in ordinary life. If you hear it once, the effect is usually mild - although it can still be devastatingly effective if it plays upon a powerful fear in that individual. The more often you hear it, the more influential that suggestion becomes in the Subconscious mind. Suggestions we hear dozens of times over many years can end up just seeming like fact. "It must be true," assumes the imaginative Subconscious, "or else why would we keep hearing about it all the time?" Nevertheless, different people will respond to the suggestion in different ways depending on how that suggestion makes them feel. For example, a person who has always been skinny without ever having to fight a battle over it has no fear of weight gain at all, so is likely to feel indifferent to the suggestion. In that case the suggestion is ignored, and is unlikely to become accepted as 'fact' so it never becomes an expectation. Since it is not the suggestion itself but the effect of the *accepted* suggestion (i.e. the expectation) which is the cause of weight gain in this scenario, the skinny person is unlikely to gain weight for that reason – although any of the other three factors may still cause it.

In contrast, a person who is afraid of weight gain or is already struggling with their weight will be highly sensitive to that suggestion, as it plays upon a major fear. The reaction to this can actually be strong enough to create an enhanced inclination to smoke – an attempt to fend off the dreaded weight gain – or in the belief that they might actually lose weight that way. Today's society being what it is - largely due to the relentless influence of fashion, and also advertising - weight connotes unattractiveness and it is women who bear the brunt of this image fascism. Therefore this fear is more common in women, and so the effect of this factor more likely to be influential in actual weight-gain in women than in men. In truth it can affect either sex but the good news is, it is easily preventable with hypnotherapy.

3. Recovering the Sense of Taste

Once you are no longer smoking, and as soon as the tar clears off the taste buds on the back of your tongue, food starts to taste the way it should, and food tastes good. Without hypnotherapy, this could cause some ex-smokers to get a little over-excited by these new taste sensations, and overdo it a bit with the quantities. With hypnotherapy we make sure you can enjoy your newly-discovered sense of taste to the full without it making you overeat. All eating behaviour is habitual and compulsive, i.e. it is directly controlled by the Subconscious, so overeating can be prevented upon request during therapy.

4.  The Subconscious "Reward"

This has to do with the way quitting is being regarded at an emotional level. When people decide to stop smoking, especially if they are *not* using hypnotherapy, they may be regarding the whole thing as a sacrifice, and probably a struggle too. If so, they may not succeed at all but if they do, it is quite common for those people to then experience compulsive urges to eat things they were not compulsively eating before, or for that kind of behaviour to noticeably increase. What is going on there is that their Subconscious mind, motivated by the sense of a 'sacrifice' being made, decides to compensate by 'rewarding' with another article, and it is quite likely to be something already regarded by that person as a 'reward' such as chocolate. This can even happen in people who don't particularly enjoy chocolate, because it is the *idea* of chocolate as a reward - not the experience of real chocolate - that is driving the behaviour. And of course, the idea of 'chocolate as a reward' was programmed into us all at a very early age. The same thing can happen with sweets, and the person may be very surprised by this as they do not usually eat sweets and don't find them especially pleasant anyway, which was the main reason they didn't buy them ordinarily. These compulsive urges are easily removed with hypnotherapy.

In some cases there is no particular reward item, just more eating. Food is a pleasure in itself to many people. So to compensate for the 'loss' of the original article, and the 'suffering' if you are doing this the hard way, your Subconscious sends you powerful impulses to consume other things. With hypnotherapy there is no struggle, and we can easily get rid of the idea that this is a sacrifice and replace that with the concept of a 'liberation', which is what it really is. Once that is properly established in the Subconscious mind, getting rid of tobacco is seen as a reward in itself, so further rewards become unnecessary.

People who have experienced the reactions detailed above but didn't understand what was really causing them at the time may have come up with spurious explanations of their own, or accepted them from other people. Remember, the conscious mind must always be able to come up with a plausible reason for everything you do. So now you are compelled to explain to yourself why you are suddenly eating other peoples' dinners as well as your own. Since the conscious mind does not know the real reason, it makes up a likely tale: "I'm doing this because I don't know what to do with my hands, now I've stopped smoking." or "I'm used to putting things in my mouth, but now I've stopped smoking." These are incorrect guesses, but they seem plausible on the face of it and most smokers have heard those things said before by other smokers, so they seem readily-acceptable notions, simply because they are familiar. The true cause is one or other of the factors listed above, and these can be easily removed by effective suggestion during trance.

All four of these causes of over-eating or weight-gain can be eliminated with hypnotherapy provided the therapist knows how to do that, of course. Weight loss with hypnosis is easy to achieve too, so there is no need at all to cling on to tobacco for that reason. There are plenty of fat smokers around as living proof tobacco doesn't keep people slim – and anyway, tobacco can damage you in truly horrible ways, so it is really just a matter of getting your priorities right, and not finding yourself losing weight for the very worst of reasons - or paralysed by a stroke, which also might affect your ability to get into those jeans.

With effective hypnotherapy, there is no need for those risks of cancer or stroke, no need for the smoking and no need for the weight gain either.

### h). "It alleviates boredom, gives me something to do with my hands."

Of all the things smokers commonly say, this is the one I find most amusing because it is such a fine example of the conscious mind struggling to remain logical.

As I have said, the conscious mind does not know the real reason the habit persists because it doesn't understand what a Compulsive Habit is. The conscious mind has been led to believe it controls everything, and has a reason for all behaviour. Therefore it feels very much inclined to produce a reason even if it doesn't know what the real reason is. And as long as it sounds fairly plausible, that will do for the time being. We have something to tell ourselves - or somebody else - so we can maintain the illusion of being in conscious control.

With the 'boredom' notion however, the conscious mind is clearly struggling. First of all, no-one would dream of claiming that chewing nicotine gum gave them "something to do with their mouth", or that a nicotine patch gives you "something to wear on your upper arm". As for the suggestion that there could ever be *a need to do something* with your hands, that is a hilarious idea. They aren't in the way and they don't need to be kept occupied. What do smokers think they're doing with their hands in between smoking episodes? Are those hands dangerously unoccupied then?

I sometimes challenge this idea in a rather brutal fashion by pointing out that nailing your fingers to the table top would be "something to do with your hands". In the long run it would be much cheaper than smoking and far less dangerous. And probably for many people, a great deal less painful in the end.

Now read that last paragraph again, and really let your imagination help you out with it. In terms of the consequences, smoking isn't really something to do with your hands anyway. It is much more to do with your lungs, your throat, your tongue, your gullet and your stomach. How do those parts of the body feel when you quit? Much better actually, almost immediately.

What is going to happen to them if you don't quit? Well we can't be sure anything will, but do you have a coin handy you can flip? Those are the odds, roughly.

Smoking isn't "something to do". Once you have developed a compulsive habit it becomes something you can't help repeating, just like biting fingernails. But as nail-biting is a simple compulsive habit - no beliefs attached - you would never hear a nail-biter telling you they were doing that because they were bored. Smoking doesn't reduce boredom any more than chewing your fingernails would. It is not entertaining, this is a deadly dull activity in itself. It is just breathing smoke in and out: it cannot make any situation more interesting, especially if you have already done it thousands of times before. The idea that performing that pointless behaviour yet again would make a person less bored is frankly so ridiculous that it is rather embarrassing that the conscious mind – the strictly *logical* part of the mind, supposedly - could ever entertain the idea at all.

Boredom does not cause smoking, there is no connection - but there is a simple reason for the mistake. The more usefully-occupied the smoker is, the less they smoke, usually. Smoking can be inconvenient because cigarettes get in the way - they are an encumbrance, a nuisance, an annoyance. But if you are a smoker, you've got to fit smoking in somewhere. So when is it convenient to fit smoking in? When you are *least occupied* with anything else. It is as simple as that. At that moment you may happen to be bored as well, or you may not. Makes no difference, you'll be smoking anyway.

There are of course people who do the opposite - smoke like chimneys when they're working, and smoke less when they're not, or perhaps smoke just as much in both situations. But these individual habit patterns will have been developed in accordance with what was convenient for them within their usual daily routines. We see smoking patterns change – quite commonly – when routines change. Exceptional cases do not indicate that something different is going on. Smoking remains a Complex Compulsive Habit, however individual or out-of-the-ordinary the pattern becomes in odd cases. Why do many smokers end up smoking twenty-a-day? It has nothing to do with nicotine levels in the blood, it is because there are twenty in a pack, and the smoker gets into the habit of purchasing cigarettes once daily.

### i). "It is very nice to have one after a meal."

This is a suggestion that has no influence over our early smoking behaviour. Most new smokers – teenagers – are not supposed to be smoking anyway, and may be doing it secretly for quite some time. We are first influenced by our peers and older children, and they would hardly be likely to say to us: "Take one home and have it after your tea – they're lovely after a meal you know." And even if they had, we certainly would have rejected that suggestion when we were thirteen for obvious reasons of self-preservation.

But nor would they have said: "It is very nice to have one behind the bike sheds", or in my case the school gymnasium. This is because it isn't very nice to have a cigarette at all, especially at first. We know that well enough at the time. But later we get used to it, and grow up enough to start going to restaurants and copying other people. That's all it is. We may also have had the regular experience of seeing an older family-member light up after meals on many occasions, creating the expectation that "this is what smokers do", so when we find ourselves joining those ranks we are likely to adopt similar smoking patterns.

After a meal you feel full and satisfied, especially if it was a good meal. *Then* you light a cigarette. The cigarette didn't make you feel that way, the meal did. The compulsive urge to light up at that point is just habitual, but once again the smoke is being associated with a pleasant *moment* – and getting credit for pleasure and contentment it doesn't produce. The pleasure of that moment is real, but it does not emanate from tobacco, and it certainly has nothing to do with nicotine. Smokers would not expect to respond in the same way to the idea of sticking a patch on after a meal, or using a nicotine nasal spray.

### j). It just goes together with a drink, doesn't it?

This is probably the most common association of all amongst adult smokers, and a very common factor in relapse. Yet the connection with alcohol is actually circumstantial and fairly arbitrary. It is a cultural thing more than anything, and the culture is changing.

As I explain here how we eliminate these false beliefs in the mind of the smoker, let me once again emphasize that it is not enough for the client to simply to acknowledge these matters on a logical, conscious level because even if the new perception is accepted on that level, if the Subconscious didn't change its position on it because it never heard it, smoking behaviour may well continue, or start up again later.

Let me just say that again:

If the Subconscious didn't change its position on it – and hypnotherapy would be required for that - smoking behaviour may continue, or start again later. No matter what the conscious mind thinks.

This conscious tendency to forget the Subconscious exists accounts for every broken resolution that was sincerely sworn in the first place - no matter what plausible, rationalised excuse the conscious mind invents later to account for it. "Yes, I was going to stop drinking tonight but I've had a very stressful day!" sounds plausible enough but it would be much more accurate to say: "Yes, I did make a conscious decision to change my habitual drinking behaviour today but I failed to realise that my Subconscious mind – which operates and controls all habitual behaviour – knew sod all about that and is so influential that puny conscious efforts to oppose the repetition of the usual behaviour would be rather like standing in the path of an oncoming train and trying to bring it to a halt with the power of thought alone."

You know the usual outcome. It's like going to a wrestling competition and declaring boldly: "My three-year-old child here will defeat you!" Poor little conscious mind.

## Two Very Different Things

Tobacco smoking and alcohol consumption are very different behaviours in reality – although there are one or two coincidental connections which I will also acknowledge. First of all, people habitually 'using' tobacco will typically smoke from one end of the day to the other. They don't *drink* from one end of the day to the other because that would seriously affect their day. Drinking *is* drug-taking, in the sense that people drink to change the way they feel, and it does. Alcohol has obvious effects upon mood and behaviour - that is why we started drinking it in the first place – and also because other people were doing it. These effects upon mood and behaviour are commonly understood, so most drinking episodes are limited to certain designated moments in the day or week when it is okay to be in that state, otherwise there can be serious consequences. Of course there will always be a few people who drink throughout the day, but the vast majority do not, even if they become habitual drinkers.

One of the reasons smoking and drinking have traditionally been associated is because of the many public places where it was traditionally possible to do both. In the UK, pubs, bars and clubs were the most obvious example but also restaurants and communal public spaces like sporting arenas and concert halls. For most of the twentieth century ordinary folk commonly drank and smoked in these places - as well as on beaches and promenades, in parks and gardens and on public transport, especially trains and aeroplanes. But towards the end of the century things were changing. Alcohol restrictions have increasingly excluded drinking from public spaces, and smoking restrictions continue to increase in both public and private locations. "It just goes together with a drink" will still seem plausible in the smoker's own home, but now that smoking is banned in all enclosed public places, tobacco becomes physically separated from alcohol in the public sphere for the first time in four centuries. This will seriously reduce the extent to which tobacco gets credit for pleasure that is really created by alcohol and the social situation. And when the smoker has to leave the warmth and the welcome of the pub to stand outside in the wind and rain puffing miserably on a cancer stick, well... tobacco's days are numbered, aren't they?

Actually people have been drinking alcohol in this part of the world for thousands of years. Tobacco is a relative newcomer, and was never likely to last because it doesn't make you feel good. Alcohol *can* make you feel good for a time but even that depends upon appropriate use because the only thing nicotine and alcohol really have in common is that they are both poisons. Alcohol may be *used* as a drug but in reality it is just a poison, and if you were to consume pure alcohol it would simply kill you. In fact the word 'intoxicated' literally means 'poisoned'. Nicotine is even more poisonous: a single drop of liquid nicotine injected into the bloodstream would kill an adult human in seconds.

However, we do not drink raw alcohol - we water it down considerably and the more we dilute it, the less dangerous it becomes until we reach the point when it is not doing any real harm at all, especially in adults. In fact in small amounts alcohol appears to be slightly beneficial to health and longevity, probably because it can reduce stress if consumed only in small amounts. Tobacco smoke can kill even in tiny quantities - not only through triggering asthma attacks but uniquely tobacco use can directly cause deaths in people who were not even smoking themselves, through passive smoking.

I am not trying to play down the dangers of alcohol by the way – or exaggerate the dangers of tobacco either. These are just facts. Alcohol certainly has its downside and it has often been said that if it had been illegal for many years nobody would be campaigning to make it legal because of the terrible damage it can cause to health and society. A great deal of crime is alcohol-related, for one thing. But actually these problems are largely accounted for by *excessive* drinking, not the light or moderate drinking most adults settle for in the end. For we have to learn how to use alcohol in a way that is manageable and if drinking becomes habitually excessive, learn how to change that through hypnotherapy or else it could result in disaster. Changing this without hypnotherapy is notoriously difficult, I know. Don't assume this is because of alcohol. It is because the Subconscious needs some guidance on how to deal with alcohol, because whatever 'health advice' the conscious mind has already had, the Subconscious has had none. It is not enough to add "Please drink sensibly" to the booze adverts... it takes more than that to adjust drinking behaviour. It would also be important to make sure that your hypnotherapist is good at sorting out drinking habits in particular, not all hypnotherapists will be.

## A Caveat

Sometimes I find myself faced with a problem drinker whose original problem was something else, but alcohol was adopted as a coping mechanism or an escape. It is not uncommon in these cases for a spouse, a parent or a sibling of the problem drinker to make the original call, book the session for them or even accompany them on the day to make sure they turn up for the session, although this mistrust is usually disguised as moral support. Sometimes the therapy is paid for by one of these other people too. All these people, including the drinker, are clueless about hypnotherapy and hoping for a miracle, and when it doesn't come in the first session – and it won't – their unrealistic hopes are dashed and they abandon the method immediately.

Then the next week someone completely different comes breezing in, amiable and lively, and explains how they'd like to change their drinking habits because they've reached a point where they are usually sinking a couple of bottles of wine every night, and although they quite enjoy that, they don't want to be doing it every day because it's expensive and a bit tough on the old liver, and they would quite like to be around to see their grandchildren arrive in this world, and never really meant to do themselves any harm anyway. And I know for sure that my every suggestion to that person's Subconscious mind will be wholeheartedly accepted on that day, without hesitation, and their drinking behaviour will 'magically' change without delay, and stay changed, often without any further sessions being required on that issue.

Does that mean I couldn't help the other guy, who was more or less dragged into therapy? No, it simply means that I couldn't do it in a single session: there were too many problems and that client would need far more therapy than either of those people realised, or were prepared to invest time and money in, despite the fact it might save the guy's life. In the second scenario, the habit itself was the only thing we needed to adjust - that person made the decision for themselves and they were quite happy to change, it was what they wanted. The difference in the way that person feels about themselves and about having therapy, and the way the other guy feels about those things is so marked as to make that a completely different kettle of fish, even though they are ostensibly presenting with 'the same problem'.

In truth, the more troubled of the two clients described above has many problems, but didn't come to hypnotherapy to deal with them all – or indeed any of them. He only came because someone else dreamed of a quick fix that just does not exist in that type of case, and instead of adjusting to the reality of the ways hypnotherapy can be used to fix all those problems in the long run, the knee-jerk reaction to discovering there is no instant remedy is to abandon the method as if it were no use.

So it can be seen that quick fixes only happen in uncomplicated cases where drinking habits are concerned... but the fact is that most people who just want to adjust their drinking behaviour *are* uncomplicated cases. It has simply become habitual in many cases - drink isn't masking a hatred of their schizophrenic father or anything like that. Any problem drinker who has more in common with the other fellow should be aware that they will need to invest more time and money, but it will be well worth it if they can manage that, provided they find a good hypnotherapist of course.

With alcohol it is enough to get rid of the *excessive* drinking, there is no need (for most people) to stop altogether. And indeed many of my clients prefer not to be teetotal - they just don't want to kill themselves with it. If you have been previously given to understand that anyone who drinks to excess is an 'alcoholic' and has to quit forever and attend A.A. meetings for the rest of their lives, please be assured that whoever told you that knows nothing about the Subconscious mind. Any attempts to quit or cut down habitual drinking *without* talking to the Subconscious is usually going to be unsuccessful, because old habits die hard if you try to do it the traditional way. Returning to safe levels of drinking in uncomplicated cases is a pretty simple Subconscious learning process with most drinkers, who just got a bit over-enthusiastic and fell into habits that were potentially harmful in the long run. Since they don't mind changing, their mind will adopt the change without delay. Some clients will need to back this up with more session-time later, and some will not. It is impossible to guess which in advance.

## Back to Tobacco

Whatever you learn about tobacco – on a conscious or Subconscious level - there is no safe way to smoke, and no level of consumption that is unlikely to harm you. Half a century ago there was such a medical term as "excessive smoking", but that expression is unthinkable now, as it implies there is such a thing as smoking which is not excessive, but normal. Since tobacco smoking has never been normal behaviour, and especially since we now know that even passive smoking can kill people, all tobacco smoking is now properly regarded as simply damaging, unnatural and unnecessary. Not quite everyone realises it yet, but it is also completely pointless, which you could never really say about alcohol, or any of the other substances people sometimes use to change the way they feel, just for a buzz. Those things might be risky, but there is a point, which is to enjoy the altered state.

So those things all function as recreational drugs: they cause an altered state, and the aim is to enjoy the altered state. This will affect your perceptions and your judgement to some degree, so it is best not to drive, operate machinery, go out to sea on a pedalo or take the controls of a jumbo jet whilst those substances are having their effect. But no-one would suggest it is risky to do any of those things after smoking a cigarette, and of course they would be right, because it wouldn't change your behaviour or your perceptions at all, as long as you were accustomed to inhaling all those poisons.

So next time a smoker says: "It's a drink in one hand and a cigarette in the other, isn't it?" you will know that in reality those things are like chalk and cheese, and that if this person appears to be enjoying their evening it may have something to do with the drink they have in their hand but it has nothing to do with the cancer-stick in the other. That is just an old habit of breathing smoke in and out, which was masquerading as a pleasure from Day One – very unconvincingly on that day, in fact. You will also know that even if they drink a bit more than their doctor would advise, they probably won't be killed by alcohol because statistically, only a minority of them will - usually the ones that drink even more than their doctor. But in the case of tobacco, that risk of fatality rockets to about 50%. Roughly half the people who smoke habitually will end up a smoking-related death statistic if they do not stop - a level of risk equivalent to the toss of a coin.

So if you feel that your life and your future are worth more than the toss of a coin, it is well worth re-evaluating this supposed connection between alcohol and tobacco. Shall we begin that now?

## How it Started

The first link forged in the mind between alcohol and tobacco happens long before we ever drink or smoke. The first thing we know about either of these things is that we are not allowed to touch them. Long before we understand what they are, we know we cannot have them because they are grown-up things. So they are linked by that arbitrary fact immediately, and are placed in the same category in the mind - Grown-Up Stuff. Forbidden. Do not touch.

Not that we are bothered about that when we are young. Kids are more interested in their own needs and wishes, and those things do not figure in any of that. We might be mildly curious, but that is all. In childhood we might sneak a sample at some point, but of course smoke and alcoholic drinks are both revolting to children and we are very likely to conclude that we are missing nothing, especially if we only taste the drink, and so never experience any of alcohol's effects.

When we reach puberty we reconsider adult things, and this is when most people who later develop smoking and drinking habits will start to explore these things in more depth. Our experiments become bolder and more persistent, and so we may learn to smoke, and later accidentally turn that into a habit simply through falling into predictable daily patterns. Since smoking is not drug-taking – it doesn't alter our normal perceptions or our behaviour – it is easily incorporated into the daily routine, usually in between activities, so these smoking episodes are usually regarded by the smoker as 'breaks'. Thus smoking habits are commonly spread throughout the day and evening, with a long gap during the 'sleep' phase, whether the smoker is actually asleep or not.

We may also learn to drink, but in a very different way. Learning to handle alcohol is nowhere near as easy as learning to smoke cigarettes. The first thing we have to learn is how to drink alcoholic drinks without grimacing, because prior to that we only drank things that tasted sweet or fruity. Alcohol tastes foul and the stronger the drink is the fouler it tastes, especially at first. Later on we get used to that and can even come to believe we 'like' the taste, but really we are just associating the taste with the effect. If the manufacturer could produce a version of the same drink that tasted identical but had no effect at all, we would be very unlikely to switch from the old version to the new one, even if it was cheaper. And despite the fact it would be safer and healthier. We would almost certainly stick with the old one because that *does something*. So it can be seen that the taste becomes a matter of very little import to most drinkers in reality.

No, the thing that is really difficult to learn is how to drink enough but not too much - how to avoid becoming paralytic, how to avoid throwing up and embarrassing yourself in a hundred different ways because alcohol can have astonishing effects upon human behaviour. Well, astonishing at first. After a few years you've seen it all and then it just becomes annoying, but negotiating the various states of drunkenness is a social minefield in which dignity may die a thousand deaths between the ages of twelve and twenty-two. For some, the trouble goes on much longer than that, but by twenty-two most of us have learned all there is to know about alcohol and the way it affects human behaviour, and generally manage to avoid disgracing ourselves too much, at least the majority of the time.

All there is to know, that is, except one thing: most people are completely unaware that drinking behaviour can be changed by hypnotherapy if the person wishes to change it. In cases where there is no complicating factor – like mental illness, serious emotional disturbances, abuse or neglect – in other words if it is just a drinking issue, and the person would otherwise be normal and happy enough, then the habit can be adjusted. Giving up alcohol entirely is not necessary if the client prefers not to become teetotal.

This is not the case with tobacco. In nearly all cases, if the client smokes again after the hypnotherapy – even if they only have one drag of someone else's cigarette to begin with - they will rapidly return to their original smoking pattern.

Why so, if smoking and drinking are both compulsive habits? Why should there be a difference? Because drinking was always a different matter, with a different aim. It is easy to point out to the Subconscious that the 'drinking problem' was really a problem of *excessive* drinking, and mark out the boundaries of "pleasant" drinking, pointing out that if the habits are adjusted accordingly then alcohol can simply be enjoyed, and doesn't cause all that trouble. This is exactly what health advisors do when they are talking to the public, they simply do not realise they are talking to the wrong part of the mind. There is nothing wrong with their advice, but the Subconscious won't act upon it because it didn't hear it at all. Drinking behaviour is not directed by the conscious mind. Nor is it directed by alcohol. It is directed by the Subconscious, and the Subconscious can easily change it or eliminate it, whichever the client prefers. But if nobody talks to the Subconscious about it, it will probably continue repeating the habitual pattern indefinitely because that is what it usually does with habits, especially compulsive ones.

N.B. Hypnotherapy is only effective when it is welcomed. You cannot 'sort out' unruly behaviour by sending that person to a hypnotherapist if there is resentment, hostility or resistance to the intervention. Really talented therapists may be able to get around the resistance and achieve change anyway, but if the therapist is perceived by the client as an ally of the person who sent them for therapy, that can be very problematic.

Often clients ask why the Subconscious repeats damaging behaviour. The question is a logical one, raised of course by the conscious mind which has analysed the problem and can easily see the solution: change the behaviour. But the part of the Subconscious that directs repetition of habitual behaviours is not analytical, so it is not joining up the dots and connecting the behaviour with the consequences. It needs direction.

The Subconscious mind is intelligent, but it needs the right information if it is going to avoid error. Everybody understands this about the *conscious* mind - that it needs detailed, accurate information if it is going to get everything right. That is why we have education, and public health campaigns. But no-one seems to realise the Subconscious also needs detailed information, otherwise it will make honest mistakes. This is especially likely if it has also been deliberately misdirected for decades by ingenious advertising and marketing campaigns. It may then make those mistakes repeatedly, in the case of habitual behaviour – repeated mistakes for which the conscious mind struggles to account. Poor little conscious mind, it shouldn't be repeatedly called to account for things it never did. And after a few appropriate explanations, the Subconscious won't do it either. It doesn't *intend* to get anything wrong.

## A Small Sub-Group

So there is a world of difference between alcohol and tobacco, and in reality there always was. The people who associate them most closely are the ones who started smoking for the first time whilst under the effects of alcohol, because even the experience of smoking is different then. The presence of alcohol in the blood actually makes for a different initial smoking experience – too dizzying for some, but more like a drug experience for others. This is different again from the usual associations that are common in smokers, because for these particular smokers there never was a sickening 'behind the bike sheds' experience. They were feeling no pain before they lit that first cigarette, and the combined effect then makes their first smoking experience quite different from the typical one. Without the alcohol, it would simply be sickening and unpleasant.

Alcohol consumption can be usefully adjusted with hypnotherapy and is unlikely to change back to the old habits because the Subconscious can easily understand the benefits of the changes, once it has been told about them. Even if old habits begin to re-assert themselves, further hypnotherapy will correct it provided there is no complicating issue that needs to be dealt with. Theoretically we could try to convince a smoker that smoking ten a day instead of twenty a day is safer, but the trouble is it isn't true. It is dangerously misleading, like "Low Tar". This brings us neatly on to:

### k). "I only smoke a bit."

There are people who only smoke one cigarette a day and have never smoked more, or less. There are also people who have only ever smoked on a Saturday night out, during which they smoke most of a pack, then give the rest away before going home. That is the extent of their habit. They are not bravely resisting any 'temptation' to smoke the rest of the time, they are not 'being strong-willed'. They just have no urge to smoke tobacco in any other context because they've never developed the habit in any other time or place. There are no cravings elsewhere, because cravings are entirely the result of developing a habit pattern, which can only be created by repetition of the behaviour. So that 'social' smoker would only get an urge to smoke on a Saturday night out.

Obviously, if nicotine really were an addictive drug – more addictive than heroin, according to newspaper hacks, famed for their strict adherence to the facts – 'social' smoking would be impossible. People who take heroin are only able to keep it occasional very early on in their heroin-using career, when it is quite new to them. More regular heroin use is hardly likely to be light use or limited to social occasions, but regular tobacco use can be because it is not drug-taking in the first place. Every Saturday night is regular, but occasional. Three to five cigarettes per day is regular, but regarded as 'light' consumption. What always amuses me is that other smokers are usually very envious of smokers who develop this pattern, when they should really be envious of non-smokers, who enjoy better health and fitness than any type of smoker, and know that they are missing nothing.

Sometimes smokers go in for points-scoring by comparing habits. The smoker who only smokes one-a-day is derided:

"What's the point in just smoking one? You might as well just give up!" This implies that inhaling poisonous gases makes more sense if you do it on twenty different occasions throughout the day, rather than just once. The twenty-a-day man will easily recognise that smoking one cigarette is completely pointless and you might as well not bother, but fail to see that the same is true of each cigarette he smokes too. He is just doing the same pointless thing more often. Heavy smokers might even sneer at a ten-a-day habit: "Of course, you're not *really* a smoker, are you? Not what *I'd* call a *real* smoker, anyway!"

Question: What is a real smoker? Answer: A person who really smokes, using their real lungs to inhale real toxic fumes into their real body.

With real consequences.

There's nothing clever about smoking, that's for sure. So to be mocking people who do it less, or hardly at all is completely the wrong way round. And there is nothing planned about the development of *any* habit, it just develops automatically according to circumstances, and conscious control is relinquished fairly early on without the smoker even noticing. It is not a matter of choice or design. So it is ridiculous for smokers to compare smoking patterns, as if the pattern implied something about what kind of a person you are, or your attitudes to life. Yet smokers often make judgements and accuse one another of this or that, based on 'differences' that amount to very little in the end. And envying people who only really have a reduced version of the same problem is a bit like a man with a broken leg envying a small boy with a broken leg, as if the leg being smaller made it 'less' of a broken leg. Obviously no-one would think that - yet a twenty-a-day smoker might well envy a five-a-day man, or an occasional smoker rather than a non-smoker!

A smoker is a smoker. You can never be 'a bit of a smoker' in the same sense that you cannot have 'a bit of a cancerous tumour'. You either do smoke or you don't. You either have it or you haven't. And smoking less won't get you a less dangerous tumour, or one that will kindly take into account the fact that you don't smoke as much as you used to. Or that you smoke less than someone else, who still seems okay. Or the fact that your mum has been smoking much longer than you have and hasn't had a tumour yet.

But you kind of hoped it would, didn't you?

### I). "It won't happen to me."

First of all, we are all familiar with the general feeling that "It won't happen to me", whatever spin we personally put on it. Generally, the attitude we attach to that idea is a direct result of the way life has treated us in the past – because what we are really talking about here are the expectations of the conscious, allegedly rational mind.

When people come to me to stop smoking, they come with all kinds of different conscious expectations which are a result of many influences. There are people who say they have decided to stop smoking because they hate the way it makes them smell, whilst cheerfully acknowledging that the health aspect of things has never really worried them (it won't happen to me). There are smokers who say that they might come back for a smoking session later, but first they want to lose some weight, because that's more important than avoiding mouth cancer (that won't happen to *me*, surely).

Then there are those who are desperate to stop, terrified of lung disease, yet expecting no success - because to them, success would be something miraculous, like winning the lottery. Nothing like that has ever happened to them before so they aren't expecting such wonderful experiences to suddenly begin at this point in their life (it won't happen to me). This expectation may still be operating even if they personally know five or six people who have been this hypnotherapist before and they've all stopped smoking (that's very nice for *them*, but it won't happen to *me*. Just *my* luck I'll be the one 'it' doesn't work on). They don't realise that this negative attitude is precisely what blocks their positive response... and then the negative result seems to confirm that the negative expectation was the correct one to have, reinforcing that attitude for later dissuasion and failure. You can see how this can become cyclical: the fear of failure and the expectations of failure chasing each other all the way to the Failure Finishing Line.

Whatever the case, the same principle is involved and it is probably the most serious limitation of the poor little conscious mind – as well as the precise reason we always expect that – good or bad – things are more likely to happen to somebody else.

The conscious mind is trained to be logical. Rational. Its function is to help us deal with the outside world and other people, negotiating our way through the present and preparing for the future. The formal education which the conscious mind receives is entirely designed to assist this project, and almost exclusively geared towards making us easily employable and able to function well within The World Out There. Not the natural world of course, but the commercial industrial consumerist world - provider of all needs, both real (occasionally) and imaginary (most of the time).

The conscious mind combines education with experience in order to guess what will happen if we do this, or that. It recognises patterns, and also creates theoretical patterns of its own, testing them out. But all of this is based entirely on what has gone before, whether education or experience. It combines the two, and where it finds corroboration of the education in its experience of the real world, it regards that 'knowledge' as valid, and *then* bases expectations upon it. Where education conflicts with experience, it tends to lend more weight to experience - provided it is the mind of an adaptable, confident individual. If it is not, that person may go on for some time blindly following the theoretical models of their education, determined to stick to that regardless of how much their actual experience invalidates it. Perhaps you know someone like that. They are literally afraid to question what they were taught because they cannot think for themselves or they have no confidence in their own opinion.

They are much more comfortable adopting the official line, because they assume that an accredited, institutional view is more likely to be right than they are. Fine students of history are not among them, for the very opposite has often proved to be the case.

Many older smokers I work with, if we get onto the subject of how they started smoking, will declare: "Well, you know, we didn't know anything about the damage smoking caused then, not like they do today!" True enough. But regardless of what people 'know' today, almost as many will experiment with tobacco anyway. Why? Because most humans do not blindly follow their education and do as they are told, they combine it with their experience of the real world to see how valid it appears to be. Nowadays, everybody's conscious mind has been thoroughly schooled in how dangerous tobacco is, at least in this part of the world. Many of them then go on to explore their own experience of it, only to find that it doesn't kill *them*. They know (in theory) that it *could* kill them, or anyone else. But for this to be accepted as truly valid - which it would have to be before any *expectations* could be based upon it - this theoretical 'knowledge' has to be corroborated by their experience of the real world.

Now, it isn't long before there is corroboration that *other people* can genuinely get sick and die from smoking, so that part of the theory is validated and expectations *are* then established with regard to other people. So the smoker is not terribly shocked or surprised by the fact of other smokers being killed by tobacco, unless they happen to know them personally. But for the logical, rational, conscious mind to generate an expectation that we are likely to die ourselves, it must base that on hard evidence. The only hard evidence we have is the past, our previous experience. Easy enough to find hard evidence of smoking killing other people, but if there's no previous experience of smoking causing *you* a heart attack, or giving *you* a fatal blood clot on the brain, then your conscious mind does not expect it to happen to you. It expects these things to happen to other people *precisely because so far, they have.*

The following rationalisation is typical of how your conscious mind assesses the actual risk to you personally:

"How many cigarettes have I smoked so far? Thousands - maybe tens of thousands. If I've smoked 20-a-day for the last twenty years, that's around 146,000 cigarettes. Say that's about twelve drags per cigarette – that equals around 1,752,000 inhalations of smoke. Am I dead yet? No! How dangerous can it be then? I've been doing this for years! It hasn't killed me so far. Perhaps tobacco smoke agrees with me, in some way... who knows? Perhaps I'm a natural smoker, just immune to it. Not all smokers die from smoking, do they? What about that woman who lived 'til she was 106? The medical people keep saying all sorts of things are bad for you, or cause cancer – and then they change their minds, and tell you something else! Okay, so smoking isn't exactly good for your health and it certainly seems to kill *other people* sometimes, we've seen that – but I'm still here, still puffing away. I've been smoking most of my life, and nothing terrible has happened to *me*. So far, so good. I reckon I should be fine to carry on for a bit – I can always quit later, if it seems to be affecting my health."

So says the conscious mind. And it will go on saying that indefinitely, because every day that goes by seems to serve as further evidence - to the conscious, rational mind - that it will not cause your death. Simply because so far it hasn't... and of course the graveyards, cancer wards and intensive care units are full of people who let their conscious mind go on like that, right up until the awful moment that it got the corroboration it was waiting for all that time. At which point – if it is still alive – the bright little conscious mind finally validates the theoretical 'knowledge' it possessed all along, and allows you - for the first time - to actually *expect* these hideous consequences to happen to *you,* not just other people. That recognition comes a bit late to be of much bloody use, but that is what actually happens in many individuals.

Now, it can be true enough to suggest that "just one more cigarette won't kill you". When you first tried a cigarette, some bright spark probably helped you get started by suggesting that

"One won't kill you", and you may well have accepted that suggestion, because it is literally true. But it isn't the whole truth. In reality it is the combination of that one, plus all the other tens of thousands that might follow that could kill you just as easily and effectively as they ever killed anyone else – regardless of what your poor little conscious mind expects. But when you first smoked a cigarette you never really intended to smoke *thousands* of the foul things, did you? That notion probably never crossed your mind at all. One won't kill you immediately, that is a fact. But it is also true to say that everyone who has ever died as a result of their smoking habit – and that's about five million people every year, globally - would certainly not have done so if they had never had that one.

## m). "I don't want to stop smoking."

One of the best advertising slogans of recent past was for Kellogg's Cornflakes: "Have *you* forgotten how good they taste?" As a way of re-launching an established brand that was pure genius, for two reasons. Firstly because cornflakes had been around for so long that most people probably *had* forgotten all about them, and secondly because of the simple truth of it – they do taste good! That is why they were so successful in the first place.

What has all that to do with smoking? Because of the way we cease to notice things. The first impression we get of something is often our strongest impression because every time it is repeated it makes less of an impression, whether it is a pleasant experience or an unpleasant one. Even quite extreme experiences can cease to make much of an impression on us if they are repeated often enough, which is why people who study certain martial arts might one day be able to smash record numbers of roof-tiles with their forehead in under a minute, even though their first attempt to break one was probably followed by a long sit-down with an ice pack and a lot of reassurance.

So maybe it wouldn't be a bad idea to paraphrase that cornflakes slogan and use it for a campaign against tobacco:

## TOBACCO:
## HAVE *YOU* FORGOTTEN HOW DISGUSTING IT IS?

Because the truth is, most smokers have. They have become de-sensitised to an experience that every single one of them found revolting the first time they sampled it. How has this happened? Through simple repetition. If you repeat a sensation thousands of times on a daily basis, it pretty much stops registering at all most of the time.

So allow yourself, now, to drift back in time to that wonderful moment when you first discovered the joy of inhaling poisonous tobacco fumes. And I do mean the moment when you first inhaled it, because it isn't until you actually attempt to breathe it in, that you really, fully appreciate the sweet delights that tobacco smoke has to offer you. When you first sucked that hot, acrid gas-cloud right down into the very centre of your being – right into the most essential life-supporting system of all, the lungs, where it could do the most harm – of course you'll remember how your whole body seemed to sing with joy at this wonderful, magical new experience and how you simply couldn't wait to do it again. Probably lit up another coffin-nail straight afterwards, didn't you, it made you feel so good. Once you'd finished vomiting on your shoes.

People who claim that they don't want to stop smoking have certainly forgotten how unpleasant it is, but that's not all that is going on. There are a number of other factors too, leading to this claim, and they all boil down to one thing: FEAR!

<u>Fear of the Cravings/Willpower Battle</u>: They expect struggle and suffering if they try to stop, because that was their previous experience. They do not expect hypnotherapy to change that, so they may still hesitate to try it even though we explain that hypnotherapy wipes all that out. That explanation does not change their conscious expectations.

<u>Fear of Losing a 'Pleasure'</u>: The idea that smoking is a pleasure has been thoroughly drilled into everyone throughout the twentieth century by the tobacco industry, and this notion is persistent despite the fact that breathing in smoke isn't nice and the effects of nicotine cause nausea.

<u>Fear of Losing a 'Crutch'</u>: It is truly amazing how many people refer to tobacco as a crutch. Smokers and non-smokers alike will speak of it in this way, despite the fact that there is nothing in tobacco smoke that is actually of any use to a human being. Certainly not nicotine, the only thing nicotine ever helped anyone do is die.

What is a crutch? It is something strong that you lean on while you get your strength back, and it supports you until you do not need it anymore. Tobacco weakens, cripples and destroys people – it isn't a crutch by any stretch of the imagination. Crutches don't kill people.

Now, if you are - like myself - rather imaginative, that last statement may have provoked you to consider an instance in which a crutch could be used to batter someone to death. Likewise, it is just about possible to imagine a shipwreck scenario in which a sailor survives by climbing upon a big wooden carton of cigarettes, but that does not validate a claim that cigarettes are a potential life-saver. The prime movers are the maniac in the first case, and the wooden carton in the second. It ain't the crutch that's going to jail, and the cigarettes won't be winning a Pride of Britain Award. So get that imagination of yours under control.

<u>Fear that you will put on Weight</u>: If smoking prevented weight-gain, there'd be no fat smokers! But this is a very major fear for some people, and if you are one of them, re-read g). "It helps me keep my weight down". Several times. Then read it again. If you're still concerned, read it three or four more times. The key sentence, I suppose, is this: As an attempt to control weight, smoking is potentially suicidal, certainly unhealthy, costly and pretty unreliable anyway – all fat smokers being living proof. But maybe not for long.

<u>Fear that you will never escape Cravings:</u> This expectation is based entirely on previous experiences of trying to stop smoking - perhaps many experiences - none of which involved expert hypnotherapy. Effective hypnotherapy entirely eliminates cravings. All of them. Gone. No need for willpower at all, no battle to fight, no feelings of being deprived, nothing. Just a wonderful feeling of liberation, health, energy and the joy of being free.

Too good to be true? If you feel that way, it is only because you are so used to the idea that stopping smoking is difficult. Which it is, if you don't have hypnotherapy because all other methods rely upon willpower. More about why willpower doesn't usually succeed in Section 12. Do bear in mind that the vast majority of people in the UK have never tried hypnotherapy for themselves. Add to that, the fact that we were all – from an early age - encouraged to believe that if you want success, you've got to try really hard! So of course hypnotherapy sounds too easy, too good to be true at first. It's a normal assumption from the skeptical, world-weary, adult conscious mind. And quite wrong, like many things we just assume – but the conscious mind doesn't know that, because we assume our assumptions are correct, don't we? Can't be doubting our assumptions now can we... then where would we be?

So the smoker assumes they are stuck with the cravings, assumes that hypnotherapy won't change that, assumes the therapist is exaggerating the benefits of hypnotherapy, assumes it will just be a waste of money, assumes it's not worth trying, better to avoid the possibility of disappointment by doing nothing new at all, and just assuming tobacco won't kill them. Because so far, it hasn't.

<u>Fear that you won't be able to Handle Stress:</u> Some stress is normal, and we can handle it easily as long as we are well, and it is not sustained over long periods. If it gets prolonged or excessive, then we may need to do something about that, but to smoke is highly dangerous. The suggestion that smoking relieves stress is the biggest lie of the lot, and also a lethal one. The

poison nicotine speeds up your heart-rate and raises blood pressure. If you are under stress, your heart rate and blood pressure are already climbing, the last thing in the world you need is nicotine. It can kill you right there and then, with a heart attack or a stroke. Nicotine puts the body under extra stress, it certainly doesn't relieve it. The trouble is, you cannot *feel* that increased stress ordinarily, because that part of it is only really affecting your cardio-vascular system. You only feel it if the combination of the two is enough to trigger a heart attack or a stroke. The one thing we can be sure of is that smoking takes you closer to that edge than you would normally be, so as far as the heart is concerned, tobacco is no stress-reliever.

<u>Fear that you won't be able to Enjoy Life:</u> This fear is also based on previous quitting attempts, and the uncomfortable memory of trying to beat cravings just with willpower, which is very difficult for most people. Hypnotherapy eliminates the cravings, so the willpower to resist cravings is no longer required. End of problem. And of course, the enjoyment of life is not a state of affairs made possible by tobacco. In fact the joys of life are considerably diminished by a smoking habit, and for many smokers finally eliminated altogether by damage resulting from the smoke.

Still believe you don't want to stop? Well, try this: if you could flick a magic switch which would transform your life completely into the life of a non-smoker, with no difficulty whatsoever right here and now – would you do it?

If the answer is yes – rejoice! All you need is a little effective hypnotherapy and you can enjoy exactly that outcome.

If you answered no – rejoice! All *you* need is slightly more hypnotherapy than the people who answered yes.

Or of course you *could* – and let us not disrespect this preference, those of us who believe in freedom – choose to carry on regardless in a cheery and philosophical way, with that undeniable observation that we've all got to die of something. Just make sure you keep up that performance right until the final curtain falls, or it can lose the cheery and philosophical air that makes that attitude seem so appealing.

## Smoking and Self-Harm: A Parallel

By suggesting a parallel between smoking and self-harm I am not presenting myself as an expert on the subject of self-harm, but since this is really a comment upon one particular aspect of smoking behaviour, I put this forward for real experts on self-harm to consider if they wish. Nor am I suggesting that smoking and self-harm are similar behaviours, for clearly they are not. But for some smokers there is a parallel in one sense - and not just in the obvious respect that both activities are harmful to the self.

Inevitably there will be quite a lot of smokers to which the following does not apply, because smokers have differing habits and beliefs. But any smoker reading this who has felt, at any time, that smoking has 'helped' them to deal with a traumatic situation may be able to relate to this.

People who 'self-harm' – for example cutting themselves with razor blades, or similar behaviour – appear on the face of it to be simply acting self-destructively or perhaps melodramatically. To a person who has no impulse to do likewise, the behaviour seems pointless, painful, unattractive and probably dangerous too. But it is not as pointless as it looks, and they are not just doing it for attention either. Although it may draw attention, that is not really the aim.

At the risk of generalising too far – and let's face it, not all cases of self-harm will be exactly the same – it is observable that these people typically begin harming themselves at a time of extreme emotional stress or distress, the cause of which seems to be outside of that person's control, or they perceive it so to be. Frustration and intense negative emotion is deflected from the 'real' cause and turned inward, and the person injures their own body - but not in a way that immediately threatens their life. This is not suicidal behaviour, although there may be fantasies of that.

No, the motivation is to do something with these intense negative feelings: to attack, but not to go all out and attack the other person or people involved in this dynamic... if indeed other specific persons are involved. That revenge impulse is repressed, but a limited expression of violence is allowable as long as it is directed at the self. The main part of this is not self-hatred, although it may be peppered with some frustration with the self. It is mainly anger deflected inwards, because the self is a safer target to attack. It is similar to the way we tend to take out our anger and frustrations on our nearest and dearest even though they may have done little, personally, to upset us. It is safer than confronting the boss with a baseball bat.

So it is to express, and thereby release a part of the emotion, rather than a straightforward attempt just to damage the body, that is the real emotional drive behind self-harm. There may be other elements in play as well, but what really turns this into a compulsive habit in due course is that the person finds – to their astonishment perhaps, at first – that there can be a huge emotional release of pent-up feelings, some of which may have been repressed for so long, and with such effort that the release is overwhelming, almost like a drug high. This is not only a relief, but forms a strong motivation to do that again at some point if the emotional tension becomes too great.

But it is the other element of that – the distraction – which is the real functional parallel with tobacco smoking. The person discovers that whilst they are self-harming, the immediacy of the pain of cutting, which they *do* control, temporarily obliterates the emotional pain of the situation they do not control. It serves as a release, a distraction *and* an empowerment, all at the same time. So however negative the behaviour appears to the outsider, this is in fact a defensive move to deal with overwhelming feelings through a process that can be stopped and started at will.

Tobacco smoking becomes simply habitual in time, and indeed quickly becomes unremarkable as an experience. But most of us who have smoked will remember the shock of that first cigarette, and the difficulty of learning to smoke. It is likely that youngsters who are particularly unhappy at that point in their lives will have temporarily 'forgotten' their cares and worries – been completely distracted from them – during the rather stunning process of learning how to breathe smoke in and out as if it was nothing. Thus the cigarette seems to provide a temporary escape from misery - not by providing a euphoric high like crack or heroin, but simply because it is a shock to the system - so at that moment, everything else is forgotten.

It is the Subconscious which is likely to latch on to this emotional 'escape route', and it may result in another Subconscious motivation to repeat the action. The shock effect of smoke diminishes quickly, but the impression - that smoking seemed to help – is already established in the Subconscious mind, which was also previously bombarded with thousands of suggestions that tobacco is calming and relaxing through tobacco advertising, don't forget.

This type of smoker may feel daunted by the unpredictability of life, or threatened by external factors, but as long as they can now 'arm themselves' with something they can carry at all times, and regularly 'use', then they are not so powerless – or so it seems to them. This feeling was then compounded over the years by more and more advertising, coupled with the fact that habitual smoking tends to be organised around breaks in the routine or work-breaks, with the obvious 'escape' or 'relief' factor of that also being partly attributed to the cigarette itself. Once this type of smoker has grasped this idea that smoking 'helps', then there can be some considerable resistance to the argument that it does not. To most smokers, a simple explanation is enough for them to reject the idea, or some may even have rejected it themselves, before I explain. But a few smokers are clinging desperately to the notion that the only thing that has got them through their turbulent life so far, is that they can always (pick up a razor blade) light up a cigarette, so the prospect of life *without* that option does not seem to them like a liberation, understandably.

This type of smoker can be very anxious about the whole idea of stopping smoking, and usually will not seriously contemplate taking that step at all, unless someone close to them is killed by tobacco, or they are already ill themselves. Self-harmers may also be found within this group of smokers, or previous self-harmers. Major anxieties about food and body-weight are also more common in this group, as are more extreme attempts to control the issue such as bulimia. It is not unusual to find that these clients are on long-term medication, or a number of medications. Often they do not sleep very well and have a tendency to put themselves down. When these smokers do decide to use hypnotherapy to stop smoking, their overriding emotion about the process is fear. They often say things like: "How will I manage without my cigarettes?" or "What am I going to do without my cigarettes?" and of course, "What if it doesn't work?"

Lots of smokers believe they *need* to smoke for one reason or another, but for most smokers these are not passionately-held beliefs, they are willing to listen to logical arguments that prove otherwise. But the smoker who has a deeply-held Subconscious belief that the only thing that has made it possible for them to get through their adult years so far is the knowledge that their cigarettes were always to hand, may find the prospect of stopping smoking so alarming that this fear will dominate the process, and there is no enlightenment from my explanations because they are hardly listening. They are waiting for the 'hypnotist' to get on with the business of 'hypnotising them, to stop them from smoking'.

So a fear is driving the decision to quit – or to be more accurate regarding these cases, the decision to go through this daunting process of *attempting* to quit – but a greater fear is overshadowing the whole scenario. "I can't imagine being without them," the smoker will often say, "because I've always known that whatever happens, I can always have a cigarette." Just like self-harm, the 'escape' procedure can be stopped and started at will by the smoker. The Subconscious fear of losing that escape strategy is so marked in these people that logical arguments about the fact that the cigarette is not actually doing anything useful at all might well be ignored at the Subconscious level, although it may be possible to persuade the conscious mind of those facts. The conscious mind is usually bound by logic, the Subconscious certainly is not.

It is true that many smokers experience a degree of this clinginess over tobacco, but it does not stop them being successful with hypnotherapy because the belief in a 'need' to smoke is not absolute. But in the cases where it is absolute – and nearly always accompanied by an expectation of failure, together with such low self-esteem that the smoker may perceive themselves as generally self-destructive, and even perhaps *deserving* of all this damaging negativity – there is a much smaller chance of smoking being rejected through the ordinary hypnotherapy route of one session or two.

This does not mean that this person – or indeed a self-harmer – cannot be helped by hypnotherapy. But when a person like this presents for hypnotherapy, they already believe they have a ready 'remedy' for their problems and they are profoundly unenthusiastic about the prospect of facing life without that option. When positive suggestion meets a profound lack of enthusiasm, guess what happens? There is no response, because there is no power in a suggestion itself. It is how you feel about the suggestion that matters, at the moment it is presented to you – that is what generates the positive response.

So why do these people present for hypnotherapy at all? Well most of them don't, obviously. But the few who do are simply caught up in a miserable conflict of fears. They don't want to face the prospect of life without cigarettes, but they are also afraid of continuing. What they really hope for in hypnotherapy... no, hope doesn't really come into it in these cases. What they *dream of,* in their most desperate moments is that hypnotherapy might just possibly do something *to* them, like stage hypnosis apparently does. Something that might make them act quite differently from the way they usually act, as they think they have seen hypnosis do on TV. A dream that maybe the hypnotist has the power to change them, in a way that they believe would be utterly beyond themselves to achieve. They will give hypnotherapy a chance - or two chances at the outside but all the time they will be asking: "Can you really help me?" and "What if it doesn't work?" focusing on doubt and failure all the way through the process, and as a direct result of that, they might be unable to respond positively at all. They don't really listen to the explanations, and find no joy in being enlightened about what is really going on. They are just waiting for the magic process in which they will be changed *by somebody else,* but all the time they are full of fear and desperation. The mood is completely wrong, and all the therapist's attempts to change the mood meet with little response.

So what do I mean by suggesting that this person could yet be helped by hypnotherapy? Well, if they only realised that hypnotherapy could address the causes of all these negative feelings and change their self-perceptions, healing their self-esteem to the point where they would feel able to recognise tobacco for what it really is, and let go of the 'need' for an escape route completely, then we could achieve success. The trouble is, that would take a number of sessions and the cost and commitment to that would be greater. Also, it might seem even more daunting to this type of smoker to consider addressing their deeper emotional issues, especially since that is not really what they came for.

So it would not be true to say that hypnotherapy cannot help this person, but rather that there is a misunderstanding of how that would realistically work, and frankly an unlikelihood that they would opt for that realistic approach once it was properly explained. The leaden mood of this type of smoker slumps yet further when they discover it is not a 'magic' process in which somebody else 'takes the problem away', but therapy which engages with realities which they don't really want to face anyway.

They may also feel self-pity and resentment that the one-session quick fix that many people experience with hypnotherapy is 'not available' to them because of their other problems. And indeed it does not seem fair, in a sense, that people who have few cares and just want to discard an old habit – lucky people, really - usually get the fastest and easiest results. But it is simply because there are no complicating factors. The more there is wrong with you, the longer it takes to fix it, obviously. And there would usually be no success with smoking cessation in these tougher cases until the emotional issues were resolved.

## "I just wanted to stop smoking..."

So how do these people react when it becomes apparent it won't be plain sailing for them? Usually negatively, not surprisingly. They may feel like even more of a failure, bitterly disappointed, suspicious - sometimes they turn hostility upon the therapist, as if they have been conned or let down in some way. Their feelings are understandable because it is very difficult to be positive when your desperate longing for magical salvation turns to a more challenging and costly reality. They nearly always abandon hypnotherapy at this early stage, as if their fears of failure have simply been confirmed.

If so, I let them walk. I never try to persuade them to do otherwise, because that would make it my fault if the situation does not improve with a subsequent session. Also I know that these people already felt a failure, bitterly disappointed and suspicious before they even contacted me, because life had made them feel that way. You cannot blame them for that, but nor should the therapist feel responsible for the negative response of people like this because the therapist does not control the client's response whatever it turns out to be. Should we work with these people at all, then? Is it fair to take their money when their chances of success with the usual process are lower?

I think so, although I'm sure some therapists screen these people out: advise them that hypnotherapy may not be the best method for them. But if a hypnotherapist does that just because they want to keep their success rates high, that is a selfish reason that is not in the interests of the client at all. Or if the therapist just does not like it when things don't go well, and seeks to avoid some of that, that too is a selfish reason. But the main reason I feel inclined to give them a chance is because there will always be a few surprise successes even within this group. No therapist has the right to judge the client in advance and assume they will not succeed, because surprises happen and we should never rule that out as a possibility for any client, even if it is a slim chance. Their life may depend on it - and even if they turn out not to be one of the successes, they haven't lost their life's savings, it's probably less than smoking costs them each and every month. So it is definitely worth a punt.

Likelihoods are likelihoods, not certainties, and things can look more negative than they really are. Look at 'self-harm': as negative as it looks, it is really a form of *self-help*. Fortunately there is better help available, and anytime they feel like it, they can switch.

# Section Twelve

## The Willpower Myth

How often have you heard someone say this:

> "You can't stop smoking because you just don't have enough willpower!"

Smokers have this suggestion fired at them constantly, and feel that they have no defence against it because they are still smoking. So even if they are a person - like Allen Carr - who knows they are not ordinarily "a weak-willed person", the suggestion grows in power and influence the more often you hear it - just like any other suggestion - whether or not it is actually being directed at *you*.

What do I mean by that? Well, suggestions can be accepted and have their full effect even when they are aimed at someone else, because the effect is caused by how you feel about the idea. So anyone who hears or reads the suggestion can respond to it. As an example: if you are watching a TV show and one character in the show accuses another of lacking willpower - even that can add to your own fears that *you* do, too! The statement was not actually directed at you, but still the suggestion finds its mark. Of course this only happens if you already have a notion that you may lack willpower, it does not affect a more confident person because their feelings on the subject are quite different. When does a fear finally become a belief? When you no longer doubt it. So the constant repetition of the suggestion chips away at the doubt until none remains.

Also there does not need to be any literal truth in the suggestion for it to be totally effective, because it is the Subconscious fear that it might be true that leads to the acceptance of the idea in many people. Many beliefs are sincerely held, but absolutely untrue in reality. A belief is really just an idea that has been accepted by the mind *as if it were simply a reality*. Of course some beliefs actually are realities, but many are not, they are just ideas that are no longer being questioned in that person's mind. Naturally we do not think this is true of the beliefs we hold ourselves, but we can easily recognise the fact when we consider the things other people believe. Belief operates like a two-way mirror: we can easily 'see through' other people's beliefs, but not our own - those just appear real.

## No Enthusiasm is required to accept Negative Suggestions

Actually, enthusiasm isn't strictly necessary when it comes to responding to positive suggestions either. As long as there is no serious objection to what is being suggested, that person might respond positively. It's just that positive change never results from a positive suggestion you really don't like the sound of, such as: "All through the winter, you'll be down at that gym for 7am every day!" (Well, I wouldn't like the sound of that, anyway. So however deep in trance I might have been when that suggestion was trotted out, all through the winter I would remain warmly tucked up in bed until 8am, not dreaming about the gym.)

A negative suggestion, on the other hand, can be effortlessly accepted even when the idea being presented is a most unwelcome one, such as this one, for example:

> "The trouble with you is, you're spineless! You'd have been no use in the Normandy landings under a hail of Nazi machine-gun fire! You'd have been cowering like a frightened puppy!"

No man likes to think that might be true, but any bloke who has never even held a rifle but has seen the movie *Saving Private Ryan* might honestly find that suggestion more believable than the notion that they would charge *towards* the machine-guns shouting: "Come on you soft bastards! Is that the best you can do?"

So however much the smoker tries *not* to accept the miserable suggestion that they lack willpower, once Quitting Attempt No.3 has come to nothing they are just about ready to believe they do. Thus the suggestion may end up being reluctantly accepted anyway, and immediately their self-esteem drops like a stone. Down, too, go their expectations of successfully getting rid of the problem.

When a smoker makes a conscious decision to stop smoking, followed by a big conscious effort (willpower), their Subconscious knows absolutely nothing about it and continues directing the usual habitual behaviour. This causes an unnecessary conflict between the conscious mind and the Subconscious. All the conscious mind has in its armoury to oppose the Subconscious is the applied effort of conscious will, and I'm going to explain here why that just will not do it for most people – and it is certainly not because they "lack willpower", that is a myth. Or perhaps I should say, a mythunderstanding.

Smokers end up believing such a notion – if they do - mainly because they are told to believe it over and over again. Many of them will finally accept the suggestion that they lack willpower simply because they do not know how to stop smoking. First they accept the misleading suggestion that they *ought* to be able to fix the problem simply with a conscious effort. Then when they find the problem isn't solved that way, they may later accept the second suggestion - that this negative outcome must indicate insufficient effort. But I often compare this to a person trying to open a combination lock when they do not know the combination. They don't need more willpower and determination, that isn't going to help. All they need is the right information, and then it's a snap. They need the right method, and willpower is not it.

Conscious efforts to stop smoking usually do not succeed for several reasons. Firstly, because the habitual behaviour is not directed by the conscious mind in the first place, so it is impossible for the conscious mind to adjust it directly. Secondly, the conscious decision to change the behaviour is something the Subconscious is completely unaware of, so it continues to repeat the established habitual behaviour, or attempts to do so. Since the Subconscious is usually dominant these conflicting forces are unevenly matched – in other words, it is not a fair fight! Thirdly, the continued application of conscious efforts to *repress* the usual habitual behaviour - by force - is hard work, which creates an uncomfortable mental conflict, so we do not enjoy doing that even for a day. Fourthly, we cannot sustain the effort anyway – as I shall explain – so as soon as we stop fighting against it, the old habit simply reasserts itself. It was only being repressed, not altered in any way.

## The Fundemental Myth about Willpower

Why can we not sustain the effort? Because of the nature of willpower itself. There is a general misunderstanding of this which appears to be almost universal, and it relates directly back to another misconception, the idea that the conscious mind is supposed to be in charge of all our behaviour and choices. If it truly was, why would we need to make any *effort* to stop ourselves from doing anything? We would simply decide to change, then change easily. But no, we have to fight a battle. What are we fighting? Subconscious-driven habits and impulses of course - which proves the conscious mind is not operating those. Due to the erroneous assumption that we ought to be able to consciously direct or correct all our behaviour however, we are led to believe from an early age that we should be able to engage our willpower in something and then just leave it like that – full on, as it were – for weeks if necessary, until success is achieved.

Now if willpower could be sustained indefinitely, that might even work – although it is still the hard way of doing it. But that is not how willpower really works at all.

## How does Willpower Really Work then, Chris?

I'm glad you asked me that. Willpower, in reality, is our natural ability to summon up an extra burst of energy – temporarily, of course – to deal with something now. Today. Something we can really get a hold of, and hopefully clear fairly soon, because we are using up a lot of extra energy to do this, we can't keep it up – at least, not for long. Willpower is quite literally an extra effort we don't normally make, so of course we cannot sustain it indefinitely.

Still it is quite useful for achieving things that won't take very long anyway. If you suddenly decide: "Right! I'm going to mow the lawn", or perhaps: "Right! I'm going to kill the next-door neighbour", willpower is quite useful then because it gets you up and running and the whole thing isn't going to take very long, presumably. But for anything that is going to go on for weeks – like stopping smoking the hard way, or dieting – willpower isn't going to do it for the vast majority of people. It will get you started, but will naturally falter some way into that attempt, as you run out of steam or get distracted by something else.

Like a cream cake.

Those old habits take almost no effort to repeat – quite the reverse, in fact, because we feel 'compelled' to repeat them, whereas willpower is an extra effort we don't normally make, and therefore unsustainable. So of course the old habits usually win out in that contest, inevitably. Then people beat themselves up because they were unable to overturn that with a temporary conscious effort? They aren't being fair on themselves, and they are misunderstanding what is really going on. But there is no need for this conflict anyway: just find a good hypnotherapist and let your Subconscious know what the problem with cream cakes is. Then a polite request can be presented to the Subconscious: can we please have all compulsive urges to eat cream cakes shut down?

End of conflict. The impulse to eat the cake doesn't come from the cake, you know. And it obviously doesn't come from the conscious mind, because we are using conscious efforts to fight *against* it.

Does the hypnotherapy solution sound too easy to you? If so, that is only because you have never experienced that kind of change personally and also because you are so accustomed to the idea that such things are necessarily difficult. Not to mention all your previous experiences of trying to change things like that the hard way.

Sometimes clients reject positive suggestions for change in hypnotherapy on that very basis, because their doubt causes them to adopt the wrong attitude during the trance. However much I direct people *not* to do this, there will always be some who do it anyway. Instead of adopting the *accepting* emotional attitude of: "Great! That will do for me – that's exactly what I came here for, this will be wonderful", they do the opposite, and all of my positive suggestions are met with a *rejecting* emotional mood, which could be put into words like this: "I don't see how this could possibly work, I mean it all sounds too good to be true – it's like my Bill said this morning just before I came here, it's all down to willpower in the end..."

Remember, there is no power in a suggestion. What matters is how you feel about the suggestion at the moment it is presented to you. That is why general enthusiasm from the client is so helpful during the therapy process; it is the yardstick the Subconscious uses in deciding whether or not to act upon this new information. The Subconscious is the emotional part of the mind, it picks up on how you apparently *feel* about the changes being proposed, which is why the client who sticks with the negative outlook might not respond.

Being negative requires zero energy, and for the kind of client with a generally *rejecting* emotional attitude to positive suggestion, negative attitudes may have become habitual anyway. Not only was Bill's negative suggestion more familiar to that client as a point of view – and therefore more 'believable' to her even though it was factually wrong - it also takes no effort to accept a negative suggestion. So even though it is quite easy to accept my suggestions, it is absolutely effortless to stick with the negative one. And we could all do that, let's face it. That's not difficult in any way. It is called "giving up", and as a strategy it doesn't work any better in hypnotherapy than it does anywhere else.

But anyone could learn to stop doing that, couldn't they? Anyone could choose to stop listening to Bill and start following the directions of the therapist at any time, could they not? In fact that is exactly what most of my clients *do* choose to do at some point, which accounts for their success. And thank God they do, or I would have had to shut up shop long ago because I certainly cannot force them to do that.

And the clients that don't? Well as I said earlier, you can lead a horse to water but you shouldn't hit it with a baseball bat, and it is the same with clients. The hypnotherapist directs the client, but if the direction is not followed, the client does not arrive at success. That is not a failure of hypnotherapy, but a failure to follow directions.

## But What About People Who Do Succeed with Willpower?

Ah, now – I knew you'd bring that up. The most annoying thing about these people is not their success – although that can be pretty annoying, as other peoples' success often can – but the way it implies that everybody should be able to do it that way. If we are going to compare ourselves to other people - and of course we are, humans are competitive social creatures – we need to be careful in our choices. To whom should we compare ourselves? If we pick somebody whom we consider enviable in some way, more admirable or successful, then we are going to feel diminished in the comparison. It is de-motivating.

Don't make yourself feel bad. You'd be surprised how many of my smoking clients have been telling themselves for years that they are "a failure" simply because (for example) their husband gave up smoking without help from anyone, but they were unable to do the same. Even if the husband is kind and understanding the wife will beat herself up about it anyway. Self-esteem and confidence are destroyed in the process, replaced by self-loathing, bitter negativity and a fear of failure. The therapist has his or her work cut out, to try to get this person out of that emotional crevasse. This is usually much worse if the husband has been using tobacco as a stick to beat her with ever since he stopped.

To put things right, it helps to begin by correcting the client's misunderstanding of what the husband actually did. First of all it is not *impossible* for conscious efforts to overturn Subconscious aims, it is just extremely difficult under ordinary circumstances in the vast majority of cases. Just how futile conscious efforts turn out to be may depend upon how motivated the Subconscious is to continue the old behaviour in the first place. A half-hearted attitude from the Subconscious challenged by a vigorous opposition from the new conscious resolution *can* lead to successful change. But it is still the hard way to do it! And relapse into the old habit is all too easy once the big conscious effort has come to an end, because the ideas and beliefs that supported the habit have not been changed by that method of stopping. So it is very easy to start again, especially since the apparent success of 'willpower' can make the ex-smoker cocky: "I can stop anytime I want to! I am in control!"

According to the research cited elsewhere in this book, only about 6% of smokers are able to stop with willpower alone. Perhaps cockiness is only to be expected - they can apparently do what 94% of smokers cannot do. But 94% of smokers cannot *all* lack willpower - that is a ridiculous idea. Allen Carr knew for sure he didn't, and so do lots of other smokers. Yet for many others it is a suggestion that is easily accepted... even though it isn't true. Willpower is simply not the way to do it. Although it is not absolutely impossible, it is *effectively* so for 94% of smokers. However this is not due to a lack of willpower. It is due to the overwhelming superiority of the Subconscious mind and its direct control of the habit, and also the fact that the Subconscious is completely unaware of the conscious decision to quit.

Even those 6% of smokers who apparently stopped with willpower alone may have had other factors helping them out. If we look closely at that small group who apparently managed to stop smoking without any help, we find that the majority of them had one or more other factors in play that would be influential on a Subconscious level, where it counts. We will come to these in a moment, but first let us consider the kind of factors that might be influential on a *conscious* level, spurring willpower efforts but having no clout with the Subconscious, such as being offered money to quit, or accepting a bet. Some well-meaning parents – having noticed that their son seems to respond to financial incentives in other matters, perhaps – will try a bit of reverse psychology and say: "I bet you can't stop! In fact, I'm so confident that you can't stop smoking I'll bet you £100 that you are not able to do it!"

Sound like a good idea? Well, I would not expect that to bring permanent success, for four reasons:

1. The quitting idea did not come from the smoker, but from the parent. Since the smoker probably defied the parent's wishes in his decision to start smoking in the first place, that is unlikely to be a welcome intervention, even if £100 would otherwise be welcome enough.
2. The Subconscious does not deal with money, and cares little about it – as we can all see from the way our attitude to money magically changes when we drink alcohol. With the conscious mind no longer making the decisions we spend it with wild abandon, much to the horror of the conscious mind when we sober up, and it has to sort out the consequences of our joyous spree. In any case, the son's Subconscious may not have picked up the details of the bet at all, since it pays scant attention to the outside world ordinarily. But it wouldn't be much motivated by money either way, even though the conscious mind certainly is.
3. The way the challenge was phrased was aimed at the conscious mind, trying to motivate the son with reverse psychology by stating something the parent knew the son would find annoying, and therefore hopefully be motivated to disprove: "You can't stop!" The trouble is, the son is wide open to that suggestion on a deeper level – being a smoker - and so probably fears it is true anyway, which makes it an easily acceptable (though unwelcome) negative suggestion. Also, the suggestion that the son cannot stop smoking is repeated three times, making it much more likely the Subconscious picked up on it, as does the emotionally forthright tone used to deliver it and the weighty influence in the son's Subconscious mind of that particular sound, the unmistakeable voice of the father. The son craves the father's approval, that is the natural order of things - but the tone of the challenge is emotionally dismissive and condemnatory. Although he may rise to the challenge on a conscious level, far from inspiring the son on a Subconscious level – where it

counts most – the father's triple vote of no confidence is far more likely to connect with all his son's most negative feelings and fears about the relationship with the father, and the effect is to weaken self-confidence and self-esteem. All of which does nothing to aid the quitting attempt. It undermines it.

4. It is all too easy for the son to convince himself that any smoking the father does not know about never happened, and the £100 might be won dishonestly. And indeed it might, but that would not produce a happy non-smoker. That would produce the worst of all possible outcomes: the damaging habit continues, and it has cost the father £100 to make a liar of the son who now resents him bitterly for proving him a failure. Even the banknotes are stained with guilt.

## Factors that Do Count on a Subconscious Level

Those few smokers who *apparently* quit with willpower alone usually fall into one of the following four categories:

a). Pregnant women This is not universal, but it is quite common for female smokers to suddenly find it much easier to stop smoking once they learn they are pregnant. On a conscious level they assume that this is because they now have a new *incentive* to stop, i.e. there is now someone else's health to consider. The fact that many of them start smoking again after the birth but whilst still breastfeeding gives the lie to that but logical conscious incentive does have a small influence – as does guilt - so it is not entirely untrue. Still, the main factor in play is that during pregnancy the Subconscious 'moves the goalposts' as it were, changing all sorts of things in support of the pregnancy. We know from our eating experiences how easily we can 'go off' something – especially if it has sometime made us ill, and is therefore now regarded as a potential threat. The Subconscious can turn the pregnant woman off tobacco smoke by weakening or eliminating the craving signal, and even raising 'disgust' feelings so that it suddenly becomes a lot easier to cut it out or dramatically reduce consumption. This is not willpower, it is protective instinct. The body has become the incubator of the unborn child, and must not be contaminated.

I do not mean to suggest this happens to all women, it does not. And some women notice that this factor is not necessarily the same in each pregnancy. It might seem really easy to give up one time, but scarcely any easier the next. Inconsistency is an attribute common to the conscious mind and the Subconscious mind alike.

Some women quit during pregnancy and stay stopped, although they might not always find that easy. The ideas and beliefs that supported the habit are unaffected, so if they used to believe they enjoyed smoking, they may feel deprived at times. Or if they used to feel as if smoking helped them deal with stress, the urge to smoke may return on a bad day.

This can of course cause relapse, but even if it doesn't, it can cause a different problem that can affect other smokers. Ex-smokers who still experience cravings months or years after they stopped, often tell smokers all about it – usually exaggerating the extent of it in the process - which horrifies the smoker and puts them off quitting attempts even more. The smoker cannot imagine a worse scenario than going through a difficult quitting process, yet still wanting to smoke for years afterwards. In the smoker's imagination this is a much worse scenario than the actual experiences of the ex-smoker, because it is inflated by fear. In truth those moments are quite few and far between, because the ex-smoker who stopped years ago will rarely think of smoking at all normally, and not be much troubled by those thoughts anyway otherwise they would have started again, obviously. There may be the odd exception to that, but that would be the norm for most ex-smokers. And besides, all these risks and conflicts can be wiped out with hypnotherapy easily.

### b). People who are so stubborn that once they have told everybody that they have stopped smoking, nothing would make them smoke.

They are usually men, but not always. You may know someone like this. They simply cannot bear to be wrong, or seen to fail in anything. This is not will power, it is *pride* – not traditionally a virtue. But sometimes these dubious emotions can prove useful, and pride helping a person to stop smoking is a good enough example of that.

The trouble is, the ex-smoker will be absolutely convinced they did it with willpower alone, which will probably make them insufferably judgemental about people who are still smoking. This can end up making a spouse, or close family member bitterly hopeless about their own quitting attempts, as the proud person will rub their nose in it, using any difficulties or abandoned attempts they experience to feed his inflated pride: "You just haven't got enough willpower, that's what it is! I stopped - just like that! I just decided: "Right! That's it, I'm not buying them anymore!" ...and that was it, I've never had a cigarette since! You just have to be determined, and strong. You're weak-willed, that's your problem."

No mate: you're just a stubborn git with too much regard for your own opinion which masks a huge fear of being wrong or ridiculed, and you have no respect or consideration for other people. You are the very worst kind of ex-smoker, in fact.

### c). People who have recently had a serious shock close to home

Such as watching their father die of lung cancer or witnessing another smoker having a heart attack, that sort of thing. But that is not willpower either, that is good old-fashioned fear – the most natural reaction in the world. And it might stop them smoking abruptly, for fear can be a tremendous motivator.

The trouble is you can't stay scared. Unless you have chronic anxiety, that is. Most people do not have chronic anxiety so they only feel scared in response to a particular threat. The fear is generated to spur them to react but the intention is that they should react immediately, not indefinitely. So the fear that motivates them to quit smoking before they also get lung cancer will fade, as the events fade into the past. The fear may occasionally return to haunt them, but it becomes progressively less influential over time. This makes relapse quite likely, because none of the ideas and beliefs that supported the habit have been challenged, so those can provide motivation to pick up the habit again later. And also, the apparent ease of that quitting experience misleads the ex-smoker - causing them to assume quitting attempts will always be like that, so it doesn't even matter if they do start again, they can always 'just stop'.

### d). People who smoke very heavily

Sixty to eighty cigarettes a day, that sort of habit. Obviously most of these smokers are killed by tobacco, which is hardly a surprise to anyone, but every now and then one of these smokers will simply stop, without apparent difficulty, much to everyone's amazement. Almost everybody will have heard of a case like this anecdotally: "Uncle Joe smoked eighty cigs a day and he stopped just like that!" Of course, Uncle Joe might have been a stubborn old git who belongs in category b)... but let's give him the benefit of the doubt here because most of these heavy smokers who suddenly stop and never pick it up again are fairly placid people who are certainly not motivated by that unpleasant kind of pride.

What motivates them to just drop it then, after smoking so many cigarettes for years on end? Well I'm going to be absolutely honest and say I'm not sure – and of course they may not have a collective motivation that makes them a category in that sense. But I do suspect that *disgust* may be the common motivator. Smoking is universally acknowledged as a disgusting experience initially, and throughout a smoker's life there will be moments when that feeling of disgust hits them again – even though it might not bother them much the rest of the time. When they are ill perhaps, or have a hangover. When they have, in their own estimation "smoked too much". When I was a smoker the most I could ever manage was about twenty a day, and I would often notice how horrible it was when I was smoking at that rate. I would eat or drink all sorts of things to get the taste out of my mouth and my lungs were feeling it too. Sometimes I was having trouble breathing. Just walking up a staircase could make me feel as if I was really exerting myself, and I often had moments when I felt exhausted, faint or queasy.

Now multiply all that by four, and you have the daily experience of a person smoking eighty a day. It wouldn't be surprising if a few of them just woke up one day and could not face it anymore. But then that would not be willpower either - just the natural disinclination to continue inhaling the fumes from almost thirty thousand cigarettes a year, leading eventually to the habit being spontaneously abandoned out of sheer revulsion. It is perfectly understandable. What is perhaps more surprising is that many of their fellow heavy smokers manage to continue smoking 80 cigarettes a day until it kills them. Even ordinary smokers find that hard to imagine themselves doing and an utterly revolting thought.

It is obvious from all this that willpower is actually playing an almost insignificant role in the process of stopping smoking, not just for the 94% who find themselves unable to do it that way but also for the 6% who thought they had. Put simply, the idea that habitual smokers should normally be able to stop smoking by a determined conscious effort is a myth. Ironically it is a myth the conscious mind is unwilling to give up, as doing so reveals the true limitations of the conscious mind's influence. But on the other hand, since 94% of smokers cannot possibly *all* lack willpower, clinging to the myth is illogical.

Illogical, or powerless? Poor little conscious mind, how could it possibly choose between those options? It is losing status, true - but only because it was mistakenly promoted to an exalted position beyond its real capabilities by Science during the so-called Age of Enlightenment.

What shall we call the new era? Here are a few fun suggestions:

- ❖ The Subconscious Strikes Back
- ❖ The Age of Brilliance
- ❖ Now We're Really Enlightened
- ❖ It's The Subconscious, Stupid
- ❖ Let's Use 100% of Our Brains
- ❖ The Age of Superintelligence
- ❖ Now I Don't Have to Be My Own Worst Enemy Any More

Feel free to dream up a few of your own, using that powerful imagination you were born with. It's part of the Subconscious. The Imagination is the main reason humans are such a successful species. We have the ability to imagine things that have never been, and then invent them – which has made us spectacularly successful so far. Here's hoping, eh?

## Interlude: Case Mysteries No.7

I have always been fascinated by castles. When I was a child I found them mesmerising, and even now, when my young son and I are playing with those little plastic bricks inexplicably named Lego, he builds all manner of things but all I ever seem to build is castles. And mazes – I like to construct a maze once in a while but usually it will be a castle. That type of structure has such an aesthetic appeal for me, and if I am wandering around a real one (and the older the castle, the more this seems to be the case) I tend to drift into trance and feel like I'm travelling in time. Every detail that catches my eye has me daydreaming about the people who created it, the person who actually crafted that or laid that particular stone in place.

Recently I was at the ancient Cornish Castle of Tintagel, which seems almost impossibly constructed from thousands of smallish flat stones, rather like a dry stone wall. The castle is perched high on a windy headland which is actually a bit difficult to get to, but it is well worth the climb. Wave erosion of the headland over the centuries has caused the mid-section of the castle to fall into the sea, making it a particularly spectacular ruin, succumbing in the end to the most gradual of sieges.

A castle is a defensive structure of course. Humans are vulnerable like all animals, but clever, so we seek to offset our vulnerability through ingenuity. Building structures that provide protection is a part of that, as is the development of weapons. One cannot wander around a castle without thinking of weapons because of the architectural design, such as the narrow, wedge-shaped windows that are easy to shoot arrows from, but very difficult for outsiders to aim their arrows through. The drawbridge, the moat, the battlements and the portcullis – it is all about protection, and fending off attack.

These aspects of the castle are not about violence, but survival. The castle isn't going anywhere: its strength is not for invading or attacking. It is a living space, a home. The threat is out there, beyond the fortifications and the structure is really defined by the technology of self-defence.

Once when I was little, I remember wandering around a well-preserved castle with my mum and dad. I have no idea where, they were always taking us places and because I lived in a dream-world most of the time I only ever had a vague idea of where we were, and couldn't tell you much about it afterwards. But I clearly remember a guide pointing out a particularly solid structure, a tower near the centre of the castle which he called the Keep.

Now I'm not sure that I am very clear about the real purpose of a Keep, because to me, paying conscious attention to detailed explanations is a bit like holding my breath. I never could do it for very long and it always seemed to become more and more uncomfortable to sustain the effort as the seconds passed. In any case, it is not important how accurate this is, but the impression I got – which is always far more significant than the reality in *my* world – was of a castle within a castle, the central fortification, a place to escape to even if the outer defences were crumbling. If things were looking bad, there was still a safer place yet – as if the Keep were the ultimate sanctuary and preserver of life, the 'womb' of the castle as it were – *a place where no-one could get you.* The castle seems feminine to me, not masculine. For all its sturdiness and strength, it remains a domestic space.

In the Subconscious, meanings shift and change. They are layered, there can be many meanings and it can be a very subjective mix. Yet some meanings, symbols and metaphors are commonplace. Some become cliches, like when people speak of "putting up defences", "building walls" to protect themselves, or trying to get someone else to "come out of their shell". We hear tell of someone who has emotionally "gone inside and shut their door", or is avoiding reality by "living in an ivory tower".

On the outside, we may be many things. We present a facade, or have a number of different faces we present to the world. These faces aren't necessarily false - they are all part of the whole, just as the different sides of the castle are all part of the same structure. These faces are part of us, but they are not the whole, which is why we warn each other not to take things at 'face value'. Each face serves a purpose, and one of the purposes of each of them is to protect the self.

The self has many defences, some of which are more external. Consider the metaphorical 'mask' of make-up for example, sometimes referred to by women as their "war-paint". Bikers still wear a form of armour, which is practical enough but also tribal, in the sense that any bikers wearing the typical leathers can connect with one another easily even if they have never met before. When I was a young rocker I often wore a biker's jacket even though I never owned a motorbike. Useful if attacked, it was quite literally a second skin – but it was also a subtle weapon in terms of visual suggestion: I wore it partly just to look tougher, so hopefully anyone would think twice about attacking me in the first place.

Some of these external defences have been watered-down so much now that they are really just a dim echo of what they once were. Helmets have softened into baseball caps, visors have been replaced by mirrored sunglasses, fortifications have become hedges and gates, the moat is just a low wall and the drawbridge is gone, there's just a picture of a Rottweiler and the words "I live here" - a suggestion calculated to make a portcullis unnecessary. (Whenever I see one of those pictures of a fierce dog with the words "I live here", a little voice in my head says: "What, on your own? That's quite an achievement for a canine – and what's more, you're a dab hand at re-pointing if that front wall is anything to go by.") These features are no longer truly defences against all-out physical attack like the castle is, but provide a symbolic barrier which may make the person feel a little more secure behind it than they might without it.

The internal self has different levels too. We can be "well-grounded" or "high-minded". Emotionally we have highs and lows. Inner Space has many rooms, passages, gateways, staircases, halls and hiding places. There are secret passageways, cellars. Dungeons. Locked rooms. Places that have fallen into disuse. Forgotten places... but they are still there.

Then there are the new areas that are always under construction, for a life is a work-in-progress. And there may be gardens too, beautiful places that are not dark or grim but all about energy and life. Yet above all, life must be protected and the ultimate protector of the self, in my imaginary concept of the castle, is the Keep.

The Keep is where the Inner Self resides, and whenever we meet and greet new people – whatever we make of them in terms of our first impressions – we cannot access their Keep and they cannot reach us in ours. It is often said that we cannot really know someone until we have lived with them, but even then there may be things about them that we do not know. Perhaps your first thought, pondering that, may be to think of something sinister, but I was not limiting the observation to that alone. People can surprise each other even after many years of close contact, because there is always so much more to everyone than anyone knows. That includes the self – yes, people can surprise themselves as well! In fact it happens all the time in my line of work. But some people do not like surprises.

Some people do not like change. These people don't seek therapy, it goes without saying. But their friends and loved ones sometimes do. Ideally, our family and friends ought to be the most supportive, helpful, encouraging and appreciative people we ever encounter, should they not? But people being what they are, and also because familiarity can breed contempt, this is not always the case. Sometimes 'friends' and 'loved ones' can prove to be the most unsympathetic, inconsiderate, obstructive, abusive, critical, contemptuous, judgemental, spiteful, unhelpful, discouraging and mocking influences we ever have to contend with, and these influences function actively as *counter-suggestion* in the hypnotherapeutic process of change. I call these people:

## The Dissuaders

There may be all sorts of reasons why someone close to you does not wish for you to achieve positive change through hypnotherapy. There may be many possible motivations driving their urges to express their negative comments and attitudes, and we needn't get into all of that here because I am more interested in explaining just *how* their influence can torpedo success with hypnotherapy both before and after sessions, however well the sessions themselves go. It all hangs on one thing: how strong are your fortifications to begin with? And particularly, how sound is the Keep? Because any negative suggestion that gets through those inner defences *really* hits home, and can do serious damage in reality.

Now, if a person has had a reasonable start in life, with support structures that nurtured and protected them (but not too much), encouraged them to develop confidence and independence, and instilled a system of core values that helped them to socialise normally and be generally happy and positive, then their defences against negativity directed against them should be sturdy. They are not *immune* to negative suggestion: no-one is, excepting True Grandmasters of Suggestion such as myself (Winner of the Golden Sword, 2005 International Full-Contact Ruthless Suggest-Off, hosted for the first time by Italy) – but in that person's life...

OK I'll pause - I might have thrown you a bit with that one. There is of course no such competition and in any case 2005 was not the first time Italy hosted it, that was 1998. If you remember I was describing a person with a fairly sound start in life? Yes, for them, negativity is not the norm so it seems more natural to question it, doubt it - reject it as alien, unwelcome and unnecessary.

Negative comments are like missiles being hurled at the castle walls. The missiles may be of all shapes and sizes, some carrying more weight than others but the purpose of all is the same – to weaken the defences so that the inner self is more easily open to attack. The missiles may come from any angle, either at predictable moments or right out of the blue. Since individual defence structures vary in strength, the damage done by the incoming attack may depend upon how sturdy the fortification was at that moment, how determinedly it is defended, how much time there is for recovery before the next assault, how many times it has been attacked before and where its weak points lie. The trouble is, those closest to us learn where our vulnerabilities are, so that they can – if they choose – aim directly at them, sometimes with devastating accuracy.

We can all relate to this to some degree. But for some people the rate of fire is constant, daily, and may have been for years. Or even decades... so that the outer walls are gone and the Keep is all that is left, crumbling and full of holes, but somehow still standing.

Who are The Dissuaders? Anyone can assume the role, provided they are close enough to take pot shots on a regular basis. They can be work colleagues, 'friends', neighbours, people like that. But more often they are family: parents, spouse, siblings or in-laws. Parents are often the worst because they have had so much opportunity over the years to bombard you with negative comments, judgements, criticisms and unwanted 'advice' that the damage they are capable of doing can end up being catastrophic.

One of my clients used to joke grimly that in her life, I was the therapist and her mother was the Anti-Therapist. Sometimes these parents had it done to them and they are just repeating it automatically. In fact we all do a bit of that – an element of it is unavoidable – but it is the degree to which this kind of attention dominates the relationship that matters. If this is just occasional and balanced out by plenty of positive input then it may even be useful to some degree, as long as it is not aggressive.

The determined Dissuader, though, has no interest in positive input and is probably not capable of it anyway. I remember one particular case, that of Anne, a woman who was a heavy smoker – 60 a day, something like that. Her husband was the same but he had no intention of trying to quit. Anne was determined to stop because she had developed breathing difficulties and pains in her legs, and she didn't want these symptoms to get any worse. She was very uncertain about the prospect of success because she had tried to quit a few times before... but she had never had hypnotherapy, so she was hopeful.

The session went very well. Anne followed everything and understood all the points I made, and was quite excited to discover that there were good reasons why she had found it difficult to stop before, and that she was not addicted to tobacco as she had previously believed. In fact she seemed to find this revelation particularly inspiring, as many clients do. After the session she was in very good spirits and went on her way a happy non-smoker, and very glad to be free.

Three weeks later she telephoned me, full of disappointment, saying she had started smoking again and she wanted to come back. On her return, Anne described how she had gone home after the first session full of optimism, not wanting a cigarette at all and really looking forward to telling her husband Frank and her daughters, Ruth and Ellie, the exciting news. She knew that they had been skeptical about her chances of success, and Frank had been very dismissive of hypnotherapy which he described as "a con", so she was eager to prove that it had been a valid choice. But when she announced proudly that she was now a non-smoker, the girls sneered "Yeah, right mum!" and Frank just snorted with derision and headed for the door: "Two days at the outside, and you'll be climbing the walls. Once a smoker, always a smoker – that's what I say!"

Anne was crushed. She had been so excited, and wanted them to be excited too – happy for her – and indeed they should have been. Of course they were basing their expectations upon the past: Anne's earlier attempts to quit with willpower and nicotine patches. They were making no allowance for the fact that hypnotherapy played no role in those failures. This is the problem with conscious skepticism, it is always backward-looking. If there have been numerous attempts before, but no successful ones, the conscious mind cannot realistically envisage success – so the conscious mind of a negative person will often just rule it out, as if it could never happen because it hasn't happened before! By that yardstick, all eventual success is impossible. That attitude is clearly blinkered and illogical, but that's conscious expectations for you.

Seeing beyond that takes imagination, and the family applied none. They should have imagined what it was like to be Anne, how concerned she was about her health and how admirable was her determination to be positive in spite of past difficulties. They should have told her she had done well, and apologised for doubting her. The kids should have said "That's wonderful, let's book another session for Dad!" That would have been the intelligent, supportive and positive response to Anne's initial outcome. Or if they preferred to be more cautious, as many people do, they could have said "That's great! Let's see how you go on, and if all goes well, maybe Dad could have a go."

Instead they chose to be cynical, and to show it. They gave her zero credit for her effort, her positivity and decisive action, her excitement about the results or her prospects of continued success. In fact Frank's parting-shot as he left the room seemed to be directly aimed at destroying those prospects... as if he was deliberately trying to pour cold water on the bright flame of her new hope before it became a blazing beacon that might show up his own customary habits in a rather uncomfortable light.

Many smokers and ex-smokers will have had a taste of this sort of negative reaction to quitting attempts. Sometimes these comments come from jokers who just like to be mocking about any attempts at positive change. Sometimes they escape, almost involuntarily, from non-smokers who are weary of the subject because they have heard it too many times before. Sometimes they come from smug non-smokers with low self-esteem who use the fact that they don't smoke to establish some petty superiority over the smoker, and do not wish to lose this useful stick with which to beat them on every suitable occasion. Sometimes they are crude attempts at reverse psychology – often from the smoker's children – who are also refusing to risk hope again, and are angry at the smoking parent anyway for not stopping successfully before.

The vast majority of these reactions, though, are knee-jerk reactions from other smokers who do not even realise the true cause of their reaction. It is because they are scared. Scared of smoking-related illnesses if they continue, and scared of the whole prospect of trying to quit themselves. Smokers are on the back foot now, especially older ones who no longer feel immortal. More and more people are quitting, and nobody wants to be among the final few who end up with the worst of the smoking-related diseases. It is that old animal instinct, the feeling that there is safety in numbers. The more smokers there are, the easier it is to believe that you might be one of the lucky ones, and also to convince yourself that smoking is relatively 'normal' behaviour. That imaginary security is ebbing away from smokers with every passing year, and that is the reason some smokers will have a negative reaction at first when another one within their circle tries to swap sides. Not all smokers do this by any means, but even amongst the ones that don't, there can be a palpable relief when someone else's quitting attempt fails and they return to the fold. If their fellow smokers' commiserations at the failed attempt now seem heartfelt, it is partly a "welcome back".

"Once a smoker, always a smoker"? I used to smoke, as did millions of other people on the planet who successfully quit. Frank might just as well have said "Once a teenager, always a teenager" for all the rational sense it made, but the Dissuader does not need to bother with incidental details like rationality. The Dissuader knows that if a shot is aimed at just the right spot and timed perfectly, with sufficient scorn and derision, it can crash straight through the newly-constructed hope and optimism before it has a chance to set solid - before the victim has had the time to build upon that success and develop *real* confidence.

Rarely is the Dissuader satisfied with one barrage, for this kind of behaviour is not simply someone voicing their opinion. This is a deliberate attack, designed and intended to do as much damage to the attempt to achieve change as possible. Nevertheless, this was not enough to bring down the success of the first session all by itself. It took more than a fortnight of sniping, sneering, snorting and waving cigarettes at Anne to finally get her smoking again.

Smoking commonly kills people, and Anne was already unwell because of it. She had been successful with hypnotherapy, but her success was systematically destroyed and she was driven back to a habit that routinely results in sudden death, or eventual death following protracted suffering. And who was doing this? Not an enemy or a stranger but those closest to her, particularly the man she married.

I'm not judging that individual. This is fairly commonplace human behaviour and it just shows how anxious and trapped smokers can end up feeling, and how some of our behaviour can appear cruel – and may be cruel, in effect – and yet be unconsciously defensive in reality and actually a sign of our insecurity and fear. There may be other, more petty motivations too: like the fear of being proved wrong about the statement that hypnotherapy is a con, but most of this is irrational animal instinct. "Once a smoker, always a smoker" in fact reveals a forlorn unconscious hope that one day smoking will become popular again, just like in the old days when Frank started, when nobody seemed to think it was dangerous, or something you shouldn't do.

We had a second session, and this time Anne was liberated for two months but the negativity was relentless. We did a third – which I only do with smoking under certain specific circumstances – but her heart wasn't in it, and I could well understand why. She had finally given up trying to recover her health because her positive spirit had been broken.

Now maybe you are thinking that Anne should not have paid any attention to all that negative suggestion, she should simply have stood her ground and proved them all wrong. Maybe even fought back? Perhaps you reckon these are poor excuses for relapse, and that if you had been in her place family members could never have succeeded in doing that to you. You might be right, but maybe you don't hear that kind of negative suggestion day in, day out. Maybe you didn't grow up with it, and so that attitude is alien to you, not the norm. Anne did her best to stand her ground, but Dissuaders chip away and chip away, and they know exactly where the weak points are. And if they are close family or work colleagues, they may be able to attack daily or even around the clock, until it just gets too exhausting to fend off the relentless blows to confidence and self-esteem and you just want it to stop.

Only one thing will make the determined Dissuader stop. How long the former smoker can hold out against the siege all hangs on one thing, as I said earlier: how strong were their fortifications to begin with? The sad irony is that Anne was actually stronger than Frank, it's just that she did not realise that was the case. Negativity is easy, anyone can manage that. It takes no effort, no spirit or energy to be negative. It takes no strength of personality to sneer, no depth of character to pour scorn on the possibility of positive change or the process of hypnotherapy for that matter. Anyone can do that - without any insight, wisdom, knowledge or experience at all, and some people do. Naturally I hate them, but it comes with the territory.

Hypnotherapy does not wear off, nor does it rely on willpower at any time. But if you are under attack, it takes effort to defend yourself. At first it might seem easy enough, but when it goes on, and on and on... That is what a siege is. The attackers are in for the long haul and the beleaguered defenders know they won't give up..., so when the outer defences collapse because they have been the target of many an attack before, the inner self ends up cowering in the Keep with little prospect of a reverse of fortunes. And when the blows begin to penetrate those defences too, as they will eventually... is it any wonder when they wave the white flag?

## Who will call this 'failure'?

Consider this: when it comes to measuring the success of one quitting method or another, how should we take account of real factors such as this? How could 'scientific trials' ever allow for these elements and influences that affect smokers in reality? And when it comes to assessing the effectiveness of hypnotherapy in this particular Case Mystery, does Anne's experience truly count as a failure of the *method?*

No. Frank will surely tell her that it was, and Anne will probably translate that into a personal 'failure' but the truth is, it was neither. It was a determined and sustained assault on Success - the systematic destruction of it. In the case of smoking it can actually lead to death too - but there will never be a trial, scientific or otherwise. It can be very dispiriting, as a therapist, when a real success is ruined like this and you see enthusiasm determinedly knocked to pieces by others. You know for sure that your client would be in much better shape if only they were married to someone more positive and supportive but there's nothing you can say about that because that's not the issue they brought to you.

The most upsetting part about it is that the relapses are nearly always interpreted as *personal failure* by the client. Relapse is never failure in my view, and this is even more the case when that person has only relapsed because they have been railroaded into it by someone close to them who probably just felt threatened by the prospect of their success. Without that factor, Anne would likely have remained successful because she was excited and delighted with the change. In fact it took quite a sustained effort to bring that new success crashing to the ground, and I wouldn't be human if I didn't sometimes feel like getting hold of the person responsible and...

Then I have to snap out of it, because it's time for the next session.

# Section Thirteen

## Why Doctors Do Not Provide Hypnotherapy

Clients sometimes ask: "If hypnotherapy is so successful, why don't medical services provide it?" Actually the fact is that some do. There are medical establishments in the USA, Canada, some parts of Europe and even a few in the UK where some form of hypnotherapy is offered or used routinely. These are fairly recent developments, and so far medical applications of hypnotherapy have tended to be limited to specific areas like anaesthesia in surgery, the treatment of irritable bowel syndrome and natural childbirth, but gradually acceptance of hypnotherapy is increasing despite the traditional inclination of medical authorities to resist it. Also there have always been a small number of GPs who have added some hypnotherapy skills to their conventional professional training, as have some dentists.

These are the exceptions, however, which prove the rule: in general, doctors do not provide hypnotherapy because there is very little knowledge of hypnotherapy in conventional Western medicine, and it does not feature in the training of doctors. They cannot provide services of which they know nothing. The vast majority of doctors know no more about hypnotherapy than the public at large, so of course their general notions about hypnosis will be wrong anyway for the most part. Their training is in other areas, and sometimes doctors have told me in conversation that their medical training included sweeping dismissals of alternative therapies.

Now I do not want to lump all alternative therapies together, because there is no school of therapy named 'Alternative'. However, in June 2006 a group of eminent doctors in the UK got together and penned an open letter to the Chief Executive of one NHS Trust calling for alternative therapies to be excluded from the NHS. In truth the NHS had only just begun to provide such services on anything like a broad scale, but the conservative backlash came swiftly, and the twin keynotes of the written attack were: the 'waste' of valuable resources, and suggestions that research indicates negligible success rates. These doctors did not mention hypnotherapy at all – most likely because there weren't any NHS hypnotherapy trials running anyway, there usually aren't - but seemed to single out homeopathy for particular censure, as if all alternative therapy is pretty much of that nature. To use their exact words, homeopathy is:

> "...an implausible treatment for which over a dozen systematic reviews have failed to produce convincing evidence of effectiveness".

For most people, if they have no personal experience of homeopathy being effective, that statement alone would probably be enough to convince them it is a useless therapy and therefore a waste of resources. That is certainly the *aim* of the statement and the letter as a whole. Now, I know nothing about homeopathy personally except that a few of my own clients have reported success with it for one thing or another, which is merely anecdotal. What makes me deeply suspicious of the attack is that it mirrors perfectly the deliberate rubbishing of hypnotherapy I have criticised earlier, in Volume I. In 1955 the British Medical Association officially endorsed hypnotherapy as a genuine and effective form of therapy but that has never prevented medical and pharmaceutical interests from calling it an "unproven" therapy whenever it suits them to do so, as if the BMA endorsed it on a whim. In the doctors' letter mentioned above, alternative therapies generally are described as "unproven or disproved treatments". This kind of pompous dismissal needs challenging.

1. *Implausible*: This is sheer prejudice. What this actually means is that according to conventional Western medical scientific principles it shouldn't work. Yes, and it is often said that according to the science of aerodynamics bumble bees should not be able to fly. So the next time you see one fly by, do point out to the bee it is being damned unscientific. There are many examples of implausible things in the universe which science is currently at a loss to explain. We don't have to be dismissive of them just because of that, especially since science usually figures out how to explain them in the end anyway.

2. *Systematic*: This word is being used to suggest rigour and accuracy, when in fact it is exactly like the word *quality,* which in itself means nothing specific. "This is a quality treatment" implies good, but it is just a suggestion. In truth the treatment could be good quality, poor quality or standard quality. Mediocre quality. Appalling quality. How effective is a review that is 'systematic'? Well, look at the new NHS computer 'system' and guess.

3. *Over a dozen... reviews*: First of all, repeating the same skeptical exercise a dozen times does not make it any more persuasive than it was the first time, but the suggestion here is that it does. And in any case, these 'reviews' are not claiming to be new research into the results of the actual services now being provided. These are reviews of previous studies, and the crucial question is: "Who funded those particular studies and what was their agenda?" You can be damn sure the people who commissioned that expensive scientific research into

homeopathy were not homeopaths, they don't have that kind of money.

So who were they and what were they *aiming* to prove? Obviously a scientific trial can be designed in such a way that results are likely to be unimpressive, if that is what the paymasters would prefer them to be. Studies can also be conducted badly because of ignorance about the subject, as was often the case with scientific studies into hypnotherapy. Some studies are more objective than others, and I have pointed out elsewhere that if you pick your studies carefully - ignoring any that find success - you can create any kind of 'review' you require, and then make statements like this one that appears in the letter:

> "A Cochrane review of all relevant studies, however, failed to confirm any benefits for asthma treatment."

The suspicious elements here are "relevant" and "failed to confirm". Surely all studies are relevant, are they not? Who decides which studies are relevant, and which are irrelevant - the Cochrane group? And for "failed to confirm", you could just read: "successfully cast doubt upon once again, just as they set out to do, by making sure they didn't review any successful or expert studies".

Am I really suggesting that this letter is a bogus attempt to rubbish therapies that might genuinely be useful before they get a proper foothold in the NHS? Are these doctors acting out of honest professional zeal, or is this a political move to try to protect territory long held by the pharmaceutical industry? I honestly do not know whether homeopathy has consistent success or not, but I do know for certain that hypnotherapy does, especially when it is conducted properly. Yet I have shown several examples of it being deliberately rubbished in exactly the same way as this, by 'eminent' persons in the medical profession amongst others. Some of that is simply done out of plain ignorance, but it may well go beyond that because there are vast amounts of money involved in the active maintenance of that ignorance.

Now I am sure that there will be lots of reasonable and intelligent people reading this who are very interested in the possibilities of alternative therapies, but once I start hinting at dark dealings afoot within the corridors of power they feel disinclined to take such conspiracy theories seriously at all. It goes too far for them - they just cannot contemplate corruption of that nature in respectable establishments like the medical profession. But any conspiracy that wasn't able to bank upon you assuming that would not succeed for long, would it? And isn't that sort of automatic disbelief - that medical persons would ever do such a thing - the most significant factor that allowed Harold Shipman to kill hundreds of people instead of just a few? His activities were pretty "systematic". But the systems that should have found him out much sooner were not, and of course it seemed 'unthinkable' didn't it?

Is it wrong to mention Shipman? Is that rather below the belt? I don't think so, because Shipman is only one example of how the medical profession has created an exalted position for itself and then abused it repeatedly, as if doctors and scientists are somehow superior to the rest of society and their judgement worth more than the opinion of a non-medical person. We are expected to *trust* them more, because of the myth of The Scientific Way: the notion that everything doctors and scientists assert has been proven in objective and perfectly-organised trials that simply establish *truth*. As the letter puts it:

> "...our ability to explain and justify to patients the selection of treatments, and to account for expenditure on them more widely, is compromised if we abandon our reference to evidence."

Notice how the word "evidence" is being presented here as if it is simply another word for "truth". But where does this "evidence" come from? Expensive scientific trials paid for by drug companies! Are you getting the picture? Of course there is not a great deal of "evidence" created that way about the success of acupuncture, hypnotherapy and homeopathy, because the large global interests that commission 'research' are not interested in researching that, they want a product. It is an industry. They don't even want to produce a cure, these days: they want to develop a treatment, and if you have to stay on it for the rest of your life, so much the better. At the end of the day this is business, it is about shifting units. This is the kind of 'research' that gave us Thalidomide, Valium and more recently Zyban and Prozac. Those new wonder-drugs were explained and justified to patients too, with reference to "evidence". Some of those patients were left wishing they had never listened to any of that "evidence".

## Wilfully Ignoring the Empirical Evidence

Now also consider the fact that these medical authorities are quite prepared to go on wasting hundreds of millions of pounds on NRT when it obviously has no real success, as their own reports now show. Also that they don't seem to have a problem with the fact that the National Health Service has really become the National Medication Service, and that they have recently wasted billions in excess of budget on a computer system that doesn't even work properly, and you have to ask yourself "Why should we be expected to have a high regard for the judgement of the people at the centre of all this?"

"These are not trivial matters", the letter says. No - and neither were the hundreds of children's body-parts hoarded under hospitals, taken without the permission or knowledge of the parents. So when these worthy professors who have added their signatures to Professor Michael Baum's anti-alternative letter refer to the government's initiative to bring complementary therapies like homeopathy into the NHS as "highly irresponsible" they should hardly be surprised if the public raise a collective eyebrow.

## My Personal Reply to Professor Michael Baum et al

I am aware that some hypnotherapists would very much like to play a significant role in the provision of hypnotherapy services as part of the NHS, so I am speaking entirely independently when I say:

> "I do not WANT to be a part of the NHS Michael, thank you very much."

I do think that hypnotherapy should be a part of primary care because it works, and I would argue that any other therapy that works should also be a part of it, whether Baum et al are prejudiced against it or not. You don't need to do scientific trials where things like homeopathy and hypnotherapy are concerned. Since they can do no harm, just run pilot schemes alongside conventional services, allow patients a free choice and ask the users of the services to review the results as part of their treatment. If they are reviewing it positively, continue. If they scarcely notice any benefit, they will tell you this. The proof of the pudding is in the eating, not the molecular analysis.

Who could possibly be uneasy about the outcome of that, except of course the drug companies? Either it will confirm the prejudices of the thirteen apostles of the pharmaceutical industry or it will not. I think the *patients* are best placed to decide, and then we can do away with the misleading variables of 'scientific' trials and stop 'reviewing' selected old research data. No need for it.

## What's wrong with the NHS?

Don't get me wrong, many wonderful things are achieved within the NHS but it is a monster of waste and inefficiency. It has simply grown too big. In my tiny little practice I get exciting and rapid results with hypnotherapy every day, for a whole range of different issues and conditions: eliminating bad habits, weight loss, boosting confidence, removing phobias and anxieties, improving sleep, resolving emotional problems and relationship issues ...to mention but a few. I've only been doing this since August 2000 yet I'm having a great time - my practice is very busy, I have nice offices in the centre of town, I get happy letters and emails from former clients, messages of thanks and dozens of referrals every month from people delighted with their success. Many of these people only had one session, and the problem was gone. They often come back later with different issues, or their relatives and friends do, so I know their success is ongoing. Believe me, the job satisfaction is brilliant and the money isn't bad either. I don't earn as much as doctors do, but there is no way I would swap places with a doctor... do you ever hear doctors talking about their job like that? I certainly do not want to be a part of the NHS! That would not be an improvement, because then I would have some moron of a manager who hadn't the faintest clue about hypnosis interfering with my work in a dozen different ways. No thanks, guys: me and my 'unproven therapy' are doing fine here: my practice has a great reputation and is very busy, and what's more, my computer works.

This is just my personal point of view, you understand.

Do you know the best bit? All those people who have been amazed and delighted with their success after visiting me - or indeed, any other decent hypnotherapist – all they did was pop along to the office and sit in a comfy chair for a couple of hours. First we had a bit of a chat, and then they rested their eyes and relaxed for a while, just as you might do on a sun-bed, while I chatted to their Subconscious mind for a time. That's it – that is all they had to do to be totally successful. Of course, it helps that they did that *with the right attitude* but apart from that they did not need to do a thing. Their Subconscious did the rest. Isn't that a fantastic way to get rid of a problem? The key is that I knew exactly what to say to that person's Subconscious and how to present that in a way that made it wholly acceptable, but for the client it is effortless.

No wonder people tend to think it sounds too good to be true if they have no personal experience of hypnotherapy success! It *does* sound too good to be true, doesn't it? This is exactly why everybody is amazed when they experience hypnotherapy success for themselves. They don't feel as though they did anything at all, really. They certainly didn't have to make any effort. *Too good to miss* - that's what it really is. Too good to be sidelined and ignored any longer by pompous, prejudiced fools like Michael Baum et al.

So why are the health services in this country organised as if hypnotherapy does not exist? Why do things the hard way, with far less success? Did you know that you cannot study hypnotherapy at any university in the land? At this time in the U.K. there is no such thing as a Hypnotherapy Degree. That is mad! You can study psychology, of course. There are thousands of people doing that. And how many of them ever end up using that knowledge in their daily work? What are all these people studying psychology for?

## Psychology: A Conceit of the Conscious Mind

The bizarre anomaly that psychology is generally assumed to be more 'respectable' than hypnotherapy and therefore more worthy of being taken seriously is sheer ignorance and prejudice. There are some psychologists who know this because they are hypnotherapists too but there are others who talk of hypnotherapy as if it is half-baked or of little use... even risky. At my own university, where I lectured for a number of years in the English Department, there was once a psychology postgraduate who submitted a doctoral thesis entitled: "Hypnotherapy: An Assault on the Mind". Even the title demonstrates a level of ignorance and prejudice which is bordering on hysteria. I didn't read the actual thesis, because I was afraid that if I did, I would feel compelled to find the guy who wrote it and shove it up his arse... and officially you are not supposed to remove these things from the library, let alone return them to their point of origin.

## Who's Afraid of the Subconscious Mind?

This is what it all comes down to, in the end. For Science, the conscious analytical mind is supposed to be supreme. Analysis is so central to the scientific project that any suggestion that the analytical conscious mind is not the dominant player in human mental functioning - and is in fact subject to a higher mental authority that is also *an intelligence* - is automatically greeted with hostility. The way science is always presented to the public – as if Science is synonymous with Truth - requires the automatic rejection of any other knowledge as inferior or unreliable, when in reality it is the imaginary ideal of science *as objective* that is problematic.

Anyone who has bought into the Scientific Ideal is necessarily suspicious of the Subconscious, because it is *intelligence of a different nature* which is not bound by reason. It certainly understands reason, but is not limited to it. Rationalists are alarmed by that, so their tendency is to reject, deny, ignore. To act as if the Subconscious does not exist - and indeed nearly everything we are taught, from the moment we enter education and almost exclusively throughout, is aimed at the conscious mind, as if the Subconscious does not exist.

This means that scientists and doctors (and of course, anyone else who is not a hypnotist, including many psychologists and others in the so-called mind-sciences) are not easily able to distinguish Subconscious-driven behaviour from the thinking and activities of the conscious mind. Nor are they easily able to distinguish between cravings and withdrawal symptoms – two totally different things. Nor are they able to communicate with the Subconscious or work with it in any way, unless they also happen to be skilled, experienced hypnotherapists. Typically scientists make poor hypnotherapists because they tend to approach hypnotherapy as if it was a scientific procedure – which it isn't – and therefore get results that aren't too exciting.

Approaching hypnotherapy as if it was a science is rather like approaching pharmacy as if it was an art. When making-up prescriptions creativity is not only inappropriate, it could be disastrous! But when working with the Subconscious mind, if you don't get creative you won't get very far. The Subconscious mind *is* the creative part of the mind - it is dominated by the imagination. If you are not succeeding in appealing to the imagination – in other words, the human ability to see possibilities *beyond* what has already been experienced directly - then you are not appealing to the Subconscious mind at all. It is an art.

I remember reading a skeptical article once in a scientific journal, which began with the words: "I've always been dubious about hypnotherapy as a science..." Quite right, mate. 'The science of hypnotherapy' is a phrase that just sounds wrong, rather like 'the mysterious art of testing glucose levels in the blood', or 'the diabolical voodoo practice of taking someone's temperature'. Let's understand the thing properly. Hypnotherapy is not medicine: it is very much a part of the hugely complex and fantastically subtle *art* of human communication, functioning on both conscious and Subconscious levels... and possibly on a 'spiritual' level too. If you think all that can be comprehended entirely by being studied and defined on a conscious analytical level in a 'scientific' way, you are a novice when it comes to understanding inner space.

NB: When I say that scientists typically make poor hypnotherapists, I do not mean that scientists are necessarily unimaginative. At the most advanced levels in any scientific field I have no doubt that the imagination of the scientists comes into play time and again. But the majority of human beings whose daily work is science-based are not working at the wildest reaches of scientific thought, they are chipping away at something rather more mundane and methodical. So when they're working - undertaking organised scientific procedures in which the imagination is not expected to play any role - they are bound to be working in analytical mode, i.e. their conscious mind is dominant at the time. Their Subconscious is probably paying little or no attention to that activity and because they work like that most of the time, they are used to processing analytically and so they are likely to do that much of the time outside work too. This would make them poor at conducting any hypnotherapy procedure. The conscious mind does lousy hypnotherapy, because it is not imaginative but skeptical, scarcely believes in the Subconscious anyway and *certainly* denies its supremacy.

Where science has usually gone wrong in its rare investigations into hypnotherapy is to get doctors, scientists and medical people to try doing the "hypnotherapy", with little or no training - and certainly no great experience - in the practice of hypnotherapy. This is like assessing the usefulness of a new and complex surgical procedure by getting *me* to perform it! In scientific investigations into hypnosis and hypnotherapy in the past, the emphasis has usually been on the mechanics of it - how to get people into trance, and testing for 'levels' of trance - as if suggestions should be accepted and acted upon provided the level of trance is right, and if not, then that person is "not a good subject"! This mechanistic approach is hilarious to anyone who really understands the human mind, but it shows what happens if you put the analytical mind in charge of studying the Subconscious. In fact the word "subject" reveals a fundamental misunderstanding in itself: nobody is "subject to" or "subjected to" any suggestion or hypnotic procedure. We are all free to do what we like with it, whether we happen to be in trance or not.

If you want to get an accurate picture of the effectiveness of the art of hypnotherapy, it is essential to have the best professional hypnotherapists do the hypnotherapy – under normal hypnotherapeutic conditions too, not under laboratory conditions - and then get the scientists to *analyse the results,* because that is what they're good at. Analysis. Hypnotherapy is not analysis, which was why Freud was so famously ineffective at hypnotherapy and invented "psycho-analysis" instead. He was by training and inclination a scientist, and markedly un-gifted in the art of hypnotherapy. Predictably Freud concluded that hypnotherapy was of little use, when the truth was that he was simply no good at it. In his new scientific mode of psychoanalysis Freud did not work *with* the Subconscious (or Unconscious) mind. Instead he analysed it, with his conscious mind.

## Camouflaging Ineffectiveness With Complexity in the Mind Sciences

Trying to analyse a Subconscious mind with a conscious mind is like a Labrador considering a painting by Picasso. The conscious mind is not up to the job, and this routinely results in lengthy periods in 'analysis' and little or slow progress. In order to cover up this lack of rapid success, the conscious mind overcomplicates everything, inventing difficult terminology and daunting complexity. It cannot easily solve the problem, so to avoid appearing inadequate it has to make the problem seem terribly complicated by analysing and theorising endlessly. Or, it assumes the problem cannot easily be solved *at all,* just because *the conscious mind* cannot easily solve it – hence the conscious impulse to reject or ignore the whole field of hypnotherapy, particularly amongst 'analytical types'.

If you pick up a book on psychology or psychoanalysis you will not find it easy for anyone to understand, like this book hopefully is. You will not find it simply explanatory but dauntingly complex, the language intellectual and esoteric. A good deal of this is phoney intellectualism and the real aim is not to understand things clearly but to be perceived and acknowledged as learned and academically respectable. It forms the pinnacle of the fake supremacy of the conscious mind, which always has to find plausible 'reasons' for its inability to *change things* – and the more complex the 'reasons' get, the better. Of course, most ordinary human beings simply cannot be bothered with any of that because it is difficult and boring, which allows the few people who are really driven by a need to feel cleverer than everyone else to pass themselves off as learned experts. It's a bit like the old days when the church conducted all its services and rituals in Latin, just so that the ordinary people in the congregation couldn't understand it properly and would hopefully be over-awed by the learnedness and solemnity of the blokes wearing the robes.

## Forget Logical Analysis...

When I am conducting the trance part of any hypnotherapy session, my conscious analytical mind is not involved in the to and fro of easy chat between my Subconscious and the client's Subconscious, it could never cope with the depth and complexity of it. I leave my conscious mind out of it - it is rather a bystander during therapy. The conscious mind can only focus on one thing at a time, whereas the Subconscious can keep fifty balls in the air without any effort at all. My client certainly wouldn't realise it but I conduct all those conversations in trance, with my Subconscious mind firmly in the driving seat. No other state of mind would be equal to the task. External reality, that's what the conscious awareness is good at handling. Not the fantastic complexity of another person's Subconscious mind.

## Understanding the Position of Doctors and Scientists

Now I don't want to be unfair to scientists or the medical profession. I'll be pretty ruthless in striking back if they dismiss my profession but that's because I know a lot more about it than they do and sometimes people need putting straight. These people can sometimes be too quick to assume the 'expert' role, not only in their own field where they may actually be genuinely knowledgeable but also in areas where they have no practical experience and are really in no position to give an informed opinion. But each doctrine – whether it is a scientific, religious or political one - will always present itself to its new converts and trainees as The Truth, and suggest that all other doctrines are foolish, outmoded or flawed in some way. To buy into The Truth, it is required that the convert cast out all Other Doctrines, and warn against them and the dangers of entertaining them, particularly if they aim to become High Priests of The Truth, advanced and privileged within that system. That exalted status is only secure if the 'Other' is constantly beaten back – other doctrines must never be allowed to encroach upon the Institutions and Bastions of The Truth.

## A Little Bit of Eminence is a Dangerous Thing

In reality, "experts" are only *relative experts* - relative, that is, to the ignorance of others. So it is possible to be more of an "expert" in medical matters than your best mate is if you know one more medical fact than he does. This obviously does not mean you are wise in all medical things, but with just a few more facts you could certainly pretend to be, and he wouldn't be any the wiser. This principle is extended to create relative experts in this field or that, but in reality their expertise is always limited by the boundaries of their training and experience, as well as their personal intelligence and insight, or lack thereof.

As we look back through history, we often smile at what 'learned' men once believed. But inevitably they grew up revering other learned men who went before them, studied their "knowledge" in good faith and valued this learning, for it made them experts too - which often gave them status, power, wealth and influence. Not surprising then, when someone comes along and upsets the apple cart by pointing out that actually the Sun doesn't go around the Earth at all (for example) so a good deal of that "knowledge" is worthless and has to be scrapped... well, such people may have to wait a generation or two for a round of applause. By which time they are usually dead, of course. Occasionally they are even killed for saying it, which is a real bummer if you were hoping for acclaim.

Scientists don't all have the same attitude to their work, but many of them were originally attracted to science because it is a system that looks sound on the face of it – we don't believe anything that cannot be proved. That seems so reassuring and sensible in principle, does it not? The kind of principle that right-minded intelligent people could devote their working life to, and be sure it was all for the good of humankind, a worthy endeavour that simply marches confidently towards greater enlightenment.

The trouble is, in reality science gets hijacked for all sorts of purposes that are not really in the interests of the advancement of science or human knowledge but the enrichment of large corporations that can afford to fund scientific studies. Scientists may not like this but they have to make a living, and they'd certainly starve if they had to wait for complimentary therapists to hire them – or even governments, these days - so they end up compromising and working for massive organisations which just use them to further their own global interests.

The original aspirations of science were higher than that, and although advancements in technology always did go hand in hand with industrial growth and military applications also - there used to be a sense in which Science seemed to be leading the way and the other interests just followed along, opportunistically finding applications for the technology. Somewhere along the line though, that changed. Scientists are no longer engaged in some glorious intellectual endeavour for the advancement of humankind. That grand project is already a thing of the past, part of the history of Science. The modern reality is that the vast majority of scientists are owned by large companies whose only interest is the advancement of that organisation. Now they have to buy into *that* as well, if they are not going to become deeply disillusioned, and that is a bitter pill for anyone who became a scientist because they were inspired and excited by its original vision. Such a lot of science now is just petty technology - neat and clever rather than mind-blowing and awe-inspiring. Mankind has exchanged reaching for the stars for just screeching round in cars, but at least the cars now have phones, sat-nav and a DVD player for the kids so that's okay, right?

## The Impossible Role of the Doctor

Did you ever hear a doctor say:

"Honestly, I have no idea - no idea at all. Sorry."

It is pretty rare, isn't it? It is almost as if they are not allowed to say that, they have to make out that they know something about what is wrong with you even if they don't. Everybody has cottoned-on to the general catch-all suggestion "It's probably a virus", and I'm sure there are many other professional techniques doctors use to help them avoid appearing clueless about something, such as the pointless rigmarole of running tests for various other things they don't really think it is anyway in the hope that the complaint will clear itself up in the meantime.

I feel genuinely sorry for GPs sometimes because they are expected to know everything and always have an answer or a solution, preferably in pill-form because most people don't actually want to go out of their way to do anything about the state of their own health, they just want the doctor to fix it. Sometimes they can. But even when they can't, the public go on expecting them to anyway. And doctors - because they don't wish to let anyone down, probably – all too often go on acting as if they can, and then just end up doing *something else,* which they know won't help much at all and sometimes even makes things worse. As if it makes more sense to do that than to do nothing or to admit that there are limits to your expertise.

## Do Not Dare to Criticise!

When I was first training as a hypnotherapist we were warned, in no uncertain terms: "Whatever you do, don't upset the BMA." That's the British Medical Association, by the way. Why not? Because they have the ear of Government, and compared to the hypnotherapy profession are enormously powerful, and the fear is that they could potentially shut our profession down. Even though the BMA has no authority or jurisdiction over the hypnotherapy profession – and indeed has always distanced itself from it – nevertheless, if they ever took it upon themselves to regard us as any sort of a threat to the medical profession's dominance of healthcare, it could be curtains for the hypnotherapy profession in the UK, this is what we were given to understand as students. The threat of restrictive legislation hovers over hypnotherapists, and it would only take a determined strike against us from the BMA and laws could be quickly introduced that could put private practitioners like me out of business completely. Something like that is already happening in some parts of the USA.

Does that seem reasonable to you? Surely the public should have access to every useful kind of healthcare there is, and the NHS is certainly not providing general hypnotherapy services to the public so if we were prevented from doing so, nobody can benefit from hypnotherapy at all. Already we are forced to be very careful about what we claim hypnotherapy can achieve, especially in advertising. As experienced therapists we know that hypnotherapy can achieve many marvellous things but we are not allowed to tell anyone, at least about *some* of it - just in case people begin to realise they don't need doctors or medicines half the time and drug companies start to lose some of their vast profits.

Well I'm sorry, but the BMA will just have to be upset. It is time to take the risk, to have the courage of our convictions and challenge them, and the vastly expensive way 'healthcare' is provided in this country, pointing out the extent to which the drug companies are really calling the shots. Right now, tens of millions of pounds every year could be saved by shutting down nicotine replacement approaches within the NHS and using some of that cash to train good hypnotherapists instead. That is just one example because there are quite a few other areas too in which hypnotherapy could eliminate the use of medication. I don't personally wish to be involved in the NHS but there are plenty of hypnotherapists that will be more than happy to get on board with that.

Why is hypnotherapy not *already* a familiar part of public healthcare in the UK? Because there are too many powerful people with vested interests who fear that the widespread development of complementary therapies could lead to a sea-change in medical practice that would surge away from drug therapies, and they are determined to prevent that shift if they can. To hell with patients and what might be best for them, we are talking about vast sums of money here – and of course money talks. In fact it is the only truly global language.

## But the tide has turned already...

The public are increasingly realising that drugs are often not the best solution and are voting with their feet. They don't want to be on medications if there is a better alternative. People are becoming much more interested in nutrition, and the *prevention* of illnesses. Sales of nutritional supplements have soared in recent years, and what is the result? Stringent new restrictions have been brought in across Europe to curb the variety, availability and range of supplements on sale. Who asked for that? It certainly wasn't the public. Can't we make our own minds up about nutritional supplements? No, apparently we need to be 'protected' from a large proportion of those vitamins and minerals and no longer allowed to discover so much detail about the promotion of *health* – just in case we end up not needing any *medicine*.

Complementary therapies are booming in the private sector, and the tardy introduction of government initiatives to include complementary approaches within the NHS really represents a slow acknowledgement of current public opinion rather than any serious change of heart on the part of the powers that be. Week after week, there are more and more horror stories in the press about unclean hospitals, 'superbugs', medical mistakes and negligence of one sort or another, and endless claims for compensation against health authorities. The image of the doctor as the exalted figure and superior being is cracking up as the NHS system struggles to avoid breaking down altogether. Media reportage of waste in the provision of healthcare in the UK is now a common theme, and the waste of unused or returned prescriptions is only the tip of the iceberg.

## Pills for Life

If the professorial signatories to That Letter really want to avoid wasting resources all they need to look at is the vast number of unnecessary prescriptions being issued and renewed daily. Huge numbers of people put on drugs like Prozac, when all that's really wrong with many of them is that they're miserable because they don't like their job, or they're not getting on with their husband, or something like that which the doctor has no time to discuss. Problems the patient might actually address, if they weren't having their brain chemistry mucked about with. Dangerous drugs like Zyban, which aren't even necessary at all since expert hypnotherapy can do a far better job. People being put on anti-depressants when they are grieving - there's another example of unnecessary chemical interference. Since when is grieving an *illness?* It's a normal part of life! Medications should be for the treatment of diseases, not the normal ups and downs of life - what the hell do doctors think they're doing, treating grief as if it was clinical depression? Many don't, but some do, and they are quite simply wrong to do that.

How many anti-depressants are prescribed now for *anxiety?* Wrong decision: anxiety is not depression. They are both distressed states, but there the similarity ends. Anxiety reactions are generated by the Subconscious mind and have identifiable causes. These reactions can often be eliminated by hypnotherapy - sometimes very quickly, especially if it is treated early on. It's just that doctors don't know this, or perhaps don't believe it because of their ignorance about hypnotherapy itself. The widespread prescribing of anti-depressants has gone too far anyway. It now seems that doctors generally assume that if a patient isn't doing cartwheels when they enter the doctor's consulting room – if they are looking even slightly down in the mouth - they should be put on anti-depressant medication - even if the patient is not convinced that they are depressed at all. Usually these days they are asked a number of dumb questions, like: "Do you ever wonder why you bothered having kids?" or "Have you ever thought of killing yourself?" and if you score enough Pissed Off Points on this inane questionnaire you win six-to-twelve months on the latest half-baked Brain Chemical Jiggling Pill.

Personally I am very much of the opinion that if a person can tell you exactly what they are unhappy about and it makes perfect sense then they are not depressed, they are unhappy about something. They don't need medication - they need help with changing that, or else with coming to terms with it, if it is something that cannot be changed. That is not the job of a doctor, but a therapist.

## Forever Tranquilised

Then there are those never-ending problems caused by errors in prescribing long ago: people put on medications like Valium and then left on it for years. One lady who came to me for hypnotherapy had been on Valium for *fourteen years!* Current guidelines suggest no more than four weeks on that drug. Am I stepping out of line, here? Does a person have to be 'medically qualified' to comment upon things like that? I don't think so, and I feel outraged by the negligence, the harm and the waste in cases such as this, don't you? We should all be outraged really because we're all paying for it. Do you know why that poor woman was taking Valium for fourteen years? I'll tell you: because having put her on the drug, the GP was afraid of what would happen if she stopped taking it because she still seemed very anxious even though she was now on Valium. As the months and years went by, other GPs in her local group practice thought it best to leave well alone, none of them wanting to take the responsibility of being the one to try to change the situation. So they just carried on giving it to her.

This is the problem with using drug therapies for non-life-threatening conditions like anxiety, general unhappiness, or sleeplessness. Either it doesn't help at all, in which case it is useless, or it does seem to help to some degree, in which case the tendency is to keep prescribing it. That is not resolving the issue but creating a mental 'dependence' on the medication, quite apart from any harm it might be doing to the body over time. Of course it is a perfect situation for the drug company - not a cure but a never-ending treatment that is ideal for generating huge operating profits indefinitely. It creates a permanent 'not-well' status for the patient though, and is very costly for the public purse without achieving any real success in the long run.

But if a hypnotherapist can resolve that sort of problem permanently – which we often can with anxiety, especially if it is treated soon enough and has not already become a lifelong thing - without using any drugs and without side-effects, isn't that simply a much better solution for everyone? Apart from the drug companies, I mean.

Back to the lady who was on Valium for fourteen years: the Valium didn't get rid of her anxiety, by the way. She just got into the habit of taking Valium tablets whenever she felt anxious, which was several times a day. She was a very anxious woman. However, if you take Valium regularly it ceases to have any noticeable effect. You build up a tolerance, so you would have to take higher and higher doses to get the same effect you got in the first place, and of course most patients would be concerned about the possible consequences of doing that. So rather than risk it she kept the dose fairly low, which meant that she didn't really feel any benefit but became convinced she would be *even worse* if she didn't take it. So the doctor not only failed to get rid of the anxiety but also gave her another problem on top of the one she had to begin with! And what did it cost the NHS, to keep her on Valium for fourteen years? I'm sure the manufacturers were delighted, but for everyone else concerned it was a disaster really.

That lady was not one of my greatest hypnotherapy successes though. I'll be quite honest and say I didn't manage to shift her anxiety either – but I did get her off Valium, and she didn't get any worse. She was grateful for that and she sent me a card the following year thanking me for that small victory. Now some might say that I had no business doing that, and only a doctor should advise her on medication. Quite right *normally,* but they had many years in which they could have addressed the issue and instead they procrastinated, renewing the prescription indefinitely.

Should I have contacted the medical practice, liaised with them? No point, they would not have welcomed a non-medical person raising questions about their patient's medication. However politely I approached the matter, their instinct would be to defend their previous decisions, which means they would have advised my client to be very cautious about my 'interference'. That would have scuppered my approach entirely because if an anxious person is warned to be cautious they are not likely to accept any positive change. So I was in a difficult position. I knew I could help her to be free of what had become a pointless medication, and that no-one at her medical practice was going to attempt that, or welcome my attempt to do what they should have done ages ago. So I was in fact her only hope of ever coming off Valium, unless she did it herself which seemed very unlikely. Together we were completely successful with that, and of course it saved the NHS some useless expense too for the rest of that woman's natural life. But how many more people are there like that out there?

## Complex Cocktails

*"Physicians pour drugs of which they know little,*
*to cure diseases of which they know less,*
*into patients of which they know nothing."*

*Voltaire*

Sometimes people come to me with a list of medications they are taking, some of which they have been on for years. I never *ask* for this information because the work I do is not medical but some people just produce a list and there might be up to seventeen or eighteen medicines on there. Now I am not a doctor – as I believe I may have mentioned before – so I am officially not qualified to comment upon the necessity (or lack of it) for any *one* of those items. But common sense surely qualifies anyone to point out that the *combination* of all these medications has unknown implications. However effectively any one medicine has been tested for safety, I'm damn sure it wasn't rigorously tested in combination with seventeen others.

This simple fact makes this sort of prescribing experimental and unsafe – even *irresponsible,* to borrow a term from the worthy professors. How does the mixing of so many medications affect the toxicity of each of them? GPs don't know, and even pharmacists can probably only guess. What is the effect of multiple medications on the health and performance of vital organs like the liver and the kidneys? What is the effect on the immune system? It's a dangerous, unknown area for everyone including the doctor doing the prescribing... but the consequences are borne by the patient. And if they die, does anyone even question the medications they were consuming daily? Of course not, because Doctor Knows Best, even if there isn't any "evidence-base" at all supporting the safety or performance of all these medications *put together*. Remember what the professors said:

> "...our ability to explain and justify to patients the selection of treatments, and to account for expenditure on them more widely, is compromised if we abandon our reference to evidence."

There is NO scientific evidence that demonstrates multiple medications are safe because they are not tested in combination, it would be practically impossible to do so. So by your own standards, worthy professors, your ability to explain and justify such experimental prescribing to patients is out the window.

After that, it is endorsed by nothing but your professional status - and you're not even risking that: if the patient's health collapses altogether who is going to point a finger at the doctor? Family and friends are more likely to point to all the medications and say: "Look at all these, see what a sick woman she was? It's no surprise she's died, but clearly the doctors did everything they could. Probably it was all these drugs that were keeping her going for this long, but they can't work miracles, can they?"

Perhaps they are right. Perhaps they are wrong. The fact is, no-one knows and in the mad world of mass medication, deaths caused by medication are not regarded as a problem anyway unless they rise above a certain percentage. And in the case of multiple medications, who is to say which one, or which combination actually caused it? The fatality cannot be attributed to any particular one of those medications, which means it will not be attributed to medication at all.

Hypnotherapy is completely free of all such risks, as are most other complementary approaches to health and restored well-being. Maybe that's why some elements in the previous administration did not regard it as "highly irresponsible" to see what these therapies could achieve in practice.

## Don't Upset the Gods

What is so frustrating for hypnotherapists is that we are not supposed to criticize doctors *at all,* even on the occasions when we know for sure that what they're doing is totally unnecessary, or actually stupid. A talented, well-trained and experienced hypnotherapist is a far greater expert in the workings of the mind, emotional problems and compulsive behaviours than any GP - but we're not supposed to say things like that, or contradict any medical advice or we might be slapped down by the collective power of the Almighty Medical Profession. This can put us in a terrible position sometimes, forced to choose between challenging the medical advice, which we are officially not 'qualified' to do, and not helping the person, which goes against our own professional ethics. The fact that doctors often have no idea hypnotherapy can get rid of the patient's problem without medication just compounds the issue.

It's not that the medical profession is totally prejudiced against complementary therapies like hypnotherapy. On the contrary, medical people often seek my services themselves so some of them certainly are not. GPs in my area also refer patients directly to me nowadays, and not just for smoking – when they hear about exciting results from their own patients, of course they let other patients know. But these are (so far) mainly issues for which they believe they have no useful medication anyway, not issues for which they would expect to treat the patient themselves.

I am sure there are many GPs who will not disagree with the key points I am making here, although they might expect some of their colleagues to be up in arms about it. But medical people usually know no more about hypnotherapy than the public, so they are unlikely to be aware of the many other things hypnotherapy can achieve and how much money and time that could save the NHS. But again, if the BMA was perfectly able to recognise the usefulness of hypnotherapy as long ago as 1955, why should there still be such ignorance about it in medical circles two generations later?

Only recently a client of mine informed me that when she told her GP she was having hypnotherapy, the doctor blurted out: "Total waste of money! You'll be back smoking inside three months!" Not only is this very ignorant of the facts, it is also irresponsible and shows a dangerous lack of awareness about the dynamics of suggestion. Fortunately my client totally dismissed this negative suggestion, but if she had held that doctor's opinion in high regard on that point – i.e. assumed that the woman knew what she was talking about - she might have taken that stupid statement to heart... and failed. Or even failed to try. But it is the *arrogance* of the doctor's statement that is really striking. That rude and ignorant dismissal is coming from a supposedly well-educated person of professional standing, who is responsible for the health and well-being of their patient. What a let-down!

## Permission to Smoke, Sir?

It never ceases to amaze me how often clients tell me that a doctor has advised them *not* to try quitting smoking just at the moment but to wait for a later time, for one reason or another. However well that is meant, it is not good medical advice because most smokers don't seriously try quitting very often anyway, so to be advised *against* it by a doctor at any time gives them several wrong impressions:

    a. That stopping smoking could be risky, when really it is continuing that is most dangerous.
    b. That continuing to smoke can be regarded as 'medically acceptable' under certain circumstances.
    c. That the doctor apparently has no confidence they will succeed... so maybe they should just forget the whole thing.

Clearly, the doctor doesn't set out to do that – rather they are concerned that the patient may not be well enough for what the doctor assumes is the 'ordeal' of quitting. But that is an *assumption*. The potential consequences of advising a smoker to continue smoking – even temporarily - could be fatal at any moment since tobacco smoking directly causes heart attacks and strokes... which are more likely anyway if the patient is going through a stressful time. In any case quitting with hypnotherapy is no ordeal, it's easy - so doctors who are under some other impression should really get their facts straight on that one. I'm well aware that many doctors are just trying to go easy on their smoking patients but they should expect that most smokers will interpret that as 'permission to continue'.

## Don't Panic, Hypnotists!

I'm not trying to launch a new militant wing of the hypnotherapy profession here but I am aware that some of my colleagues - having read this section with horror - will already be putting their tin hats on and digging themselves a foxhole before the backlash comes. I'll be getting criticism from my own side: "You can't talk to doctors like that! They'll go ballistic... they'll have us all shut down in next to no time!" Seriously, some therapists will be very afraid of that and possibly annoyed with me for daring to speak out. But there will be others who agree with me and there will be some doctors and other medical people who would not disagree with many of the points I've made. And if those people speak up too then we can have a real debate about these matters in which everyone can speak freely. Free speech is a celebrated principle in Western democracies, is it not? It isn't conditional upon not upsetting the BMA.

After all, why should we be afraid to criticise medics when mistakes are being made? Some of them don't hesitate to spout any amount of misleading nonsense about complementary therapies whenever they feel like it, just out of sheer ignorance and prejudice. And if you look at medical history, as well as all the wonderful successes there have been some howling errors along the way because they are only human. They are not demi-gods, their texts are not holy and their beliefs are often provisional. And some of them are wrong.

## Interlude: Case Mysteries No.8
## Too Much to Lose?

There are limits to human understanding and no matter how much of an 'expert' anyone may become in the activities and complexities of the human mind, there is always going to be a boundary to their expertise, and a beyond. There are different fields too: psychology, psychiatry and psychoanalysis in the scientific realm and other disciplines outside of that which also aim to heal the mind or soul of a troubled, unwell individual. Even if a person decides to train in just one field - like psychology for example - they will find a confusing number of different 'schools' within that field, all professing a different take on human mental activity and behaviour. Needless to say, not all of them are accurate in their theoretical model of the human mind and their interpretations of human actions and reactions. But they are all inclined to think they are, and the implication of that is that other theoretical models are misconceived or inaccurate.

The profession of hypnotherapy is no different in that respect. There are many schools and many approaches to the practice of that particular art of communication, many styles of presentation and also differing theories as to what is important and how things actually work – again, they cannot all be entirely correct in every detail. So when a person begins to study hypnotherapy, they have to start somewhere and whatever 'school' of hypnotherapy they happen to choose will probably form the basis of what they come to believe about hypnotherapy, at least to begin with.

Personally I do not like dividing people into 'types'. Someone once told me: "There are two types of people in the world: people who divide people into types, and people who don't", which I think sums up the practice succinctly. Nevertheless when it comes to learning procedures that involve the studying of texts, it seems to me that some students tend to regard the orthodoxy as gospel, and others who are quite ready to question it as well as take it on board. I am certainly a questioner, and consequently I have been quite happy to discard various 'learnings' along the way that I have found in practice to be untrue, or misunderstandings. Indeed a good deal of what I know about the areas in which I specialise has been learned through experience rather than teaching, although I could never have gained the experience without the teaching in the first place. Also I have never stopped studying... I just don't take anything 'as read'.

Most people who seek my professional services know nothing about hypnotherapy, although a few know a little. This is not a problem because I promptly explain everything they need to know in order to respond appropriately and achieve success. The vast majority of clients know little about the Subconscious, and haven't had any detailed information concerning the workings of their conscious mind either, so as long as my explanations make perfect sense to them and chime with their real experiences, they are happy to be enlightened according to this 'expert' view, especially if it is going to solve their problem in short order, which it usually will. This information also provides the benefit of explaining why they could not previously solve the problem themselves, which is very welcome news to the client, especially those who had been beating themselves up about that quite unnecessarily.

Occasionally however someone will walk into my office who already believes they know all about the human mind... or quite a bit about it because they did A-level psychology or perhaps studied it at university. This is not necessarily a problem in practice, it rather depends upon how much of an expert they think they are and also how much they are prepared to question what they were taught. So a person who did A-level psychology, but regards themselves as having limited knowledge and is quite happy to listen to different perspectives, will find that they can respond easily and be totally successful because they are not sacrificing the new learnings in defence of the old ones, which had not helped them to solve their issue anyway. Letting go of the old learnings seems, to that person, very little sacrifice in exchange for success with the new approach.

But what about the person who went on from A-level to do a degree in psychology, then maybe postgraduate studies - even a PhD perhaps? What about the person who then became a practising psychologist, and spent the next ten years building a career in that field? What if that person was told, by people they respected and did not question, that hypnotherapy was relatively useless - half-baked and unscientific, possibly even risky, and that psychology was a superior approach in every way? What if that person's self-esteem is largely based upon their professional status and their specialist knowledge, and the respect they assume they command as a result of all the hard work they put in over the years to achieve all that? How could they contemplate sacrificing any of that? There's too much to lose! If the new learnings I offer that person do not coincide with the learnings that constructed their professional identity, *then they must reject them* because the sacrifice involved in accepting them would be devastating. Unless of course they were thoroughly disillusioned professionally anyway and ready for a radical change in direction. Still, it's a lot to give up.

## The Psychologist

Carla was not ready for a professional change in direction but she did seem unhappy, even during her initial telephone enquiry. She announced straight away that she was a practising psychologist, and she seemed to have a real conflict about consulting a hypnotherapist at all. In fact she went on at some length quizzing me about what "techniques" I use, which is a bit pointless since I don't really use techniques. Well, that's not quite true but the technical details of what I do are really all about the intricate complexities of language and suggestion, and so deeply embedded in my ordinary conversational style that I hardly ever think about it consciously anymore, and if I started explaining all that – well, I just couldn't be bothered really, especially over the phone.

What Carla seemed most concerned with, however, was making sure I did not do NLP. She seemed slightly hysterical on this point, as if she thought that the biggest charlatans of all, amongst my 'profession', were the people who do NLP. Now some of you may already be familiar with NLP, and if so please bear with me whilst I enlighten the other readers. Also please forgive me if I'm too brief here to do NLP justice, but hey - there are hundreds of books on NLP, and this ain't one of them.

NLP is short for Neuro-Linguistic Programming, and is a (sort-of) branch of hypnotherapy that was developed in the USA in the late 1970s, blending aspects of computer 'modelling' with the work of a truly great hypnotist called Milton Erickson. He was actually a psychiatrist, but a rather unusual one who was something of a genius in his expertise with hypnosis. NLP techniques are quite easy to learn and often effective, and this therapeutic approach became hugely popular in the USA, with the main players making a fortune writing about it, teaching it and developing various schools of NLP. It has been moderately popular in the UK subsequently, and so most hypnotherapy schools over here also teach NLP courses.

Many hypnotherapists will have done some training in NLP but some really get into it and use it a lot. Personally I am not really in that camp, but I'm not knocking it. It works. In the past I have used NLP techniques myself, and they are perfectly valid. It's just not really my style but there are plenty of therapists getting great results from it. The rapidity of NLP techniques also appeal to the stage hypnotists: Paul McKenna is well-versed in this area and so is Derren Brown – although Derren Brown would object to being called a stage hypnotist as he prefers the term "psychological illusionist". He also sometimes claims that he doesn't use hypnosis, a suggestion which we might well describe as 'sleight of mouth'.

My psychologist client *was* knocking NLP though - in fact she could barely contain her loathing of it. I assured her I was not an NLP practitioner and she eventually booked in, although she seemed in a thoroughly bad mood about something.

When she arrived for the appointment she was late and in an even worse mood, blaming my directions for her lateness. This surprised me because no-one else has ever criticised my directions before or since – not really because I have fantastic powers of direction but because my offices are pretty easy to find. Still I apologised for 'misdirecting' her, assured her that it didn't matter she was late because we had plenty of time, and she calmed down a bit.

Now, for a hypnotherapy session to be a success, it is crucial that the client *wants the session to be totally successful,* and doesn't have a problem with that in any way. Don't get me wrong, I don't mean to suggest that this lady did not really want to stop smoking, of course she did. In fact she must have wanted to stop smoking very much, since she had managed to get this far - forcing herself to consult a hypnotherapist over something she – a qualified, bona fide psychologist – was unable to achieve by herself. Her desperation to stop smoking was self-evident, but clearly her opinion of my status was well below her opinion of her own, so she had a serious problem with consulting the likes of me in the first place and was (I realised later) conflicted over the implications of success.

At first, the session proceeded normally. But after about ten minutes she started interrupting regularly to question what I was saying. Normally with a stop-smoking session I spend about an hour discussing and explaining everything and answering questions, then about an hour doing the trance part of it. By the way, it is perfectly possible to do hypnotherapy without explaining it in any depth beforehand. I just prefer to do it this way because it seems to achieve more consistent results across the board. It also helps to educate people about the true nature of hypnotherapy, which is almost universally misunderstood. I thought she would find it very interesting, but it soon became clear that Carla was not going to let me get through any of these explanations without subjecting them to rigorous scrutiny - which is fine if you've got all day, and don't need to get around to any *therapy* anytime soon. As the first hour ticked away however, it became more and more obvious that this was no longer really a hypnotherapy session. It had descended into an argument about how the mind works, and a fairly grumpy one at that.

To be honest, I had my doubts about trying to work with Carla when we spoke on the phone. She had issues, and smoking wasn't the main one – always a bad start where hypnotherapy for smoking is concerned. But unusually, she actually had issues with *me* – not personally, but as a representative of my profession. And it all culminated in her blurting out: "I just don't see how you can claim to deal with anything in one session! Sometimes we work with a client for ten years!"

Well, I just burst out laughing. I'm afraid my response was entirely spontaneous and not very professional: "You get away with that? I hardly ever need to work with anyone for ten *sessions,* let alone ten years! I mean, if you haven't dealt with the issues in the first *year,* what are the next nine years about?" I couldn't believe it. That isn't therapy, it's a sentence! And of course, it became obvious at that point we were never going to make any progress, so we agreed to abandon the discussion without proceeding with any trance-work – which would have been a waste of time of course, we had never managed to establish any rapport. In the end I didn't charge her for my time, and she didn't charge me for hers. Seemed fair.

But afterwards I felt bad at first, and kept going over the conversations again and again in my mind. I wondered if I had let her down in some way, and it was some time before I managed to work out what had really happened. The truth was, she simply could not afford to take on board a new way of understanding the mind and the rapid form of intervention that is hypnotherapy, without having to question her established view of the human mind and *therapy* – which would have entailed abandoning her professional status. Since her own concept of her professional status was in any case superior to that of any practitioner of hypnotherapy or NLP, she found she simply *could not go down that road at all* and all her questions and objections were barriers, thrown up to protect her professional standing. Why was she so mad at NLP? Not because of me, that's for sure, but because it is a brief form of therapy that very often gets results instantly, so to her it seemed a threat.

The choice for her was to either hold onto her original professional belief system, rejecting the validity of NLP and hypnosis – in which case her smoking continued, and her professional progress with her clients remained tortuously slow - or to abandon her professional identity and status, and start learning about the mind all over again.

So in the end, it panned out like this. She certainly wanted to stop smoking but not at the cost of her professional identity and status. Since smoking proves lethal to half the people who continue doing it, this means she preferred to risk a 50-50 chance of dying a horrible smoking-related death, rather than genuinely embrace hypnotherapy thus jeopardizing her professional identity. And I'll bet there are hundreds of other smoking psychologists out there who would make the same choice.

## This Is Hypnotherapy, Not Psychology

Am I suggesting psychology and hypnotherapy are incompatible therapeutic modes? What about those hypnotherapists who also describe themselves as psychologists? And could not a talented psychologist incorporate aspects of hypnotherapy into his or her work? What is the difference between psychology and hypnotherapy anyway?

Well to put it simply, psychologists and psychotherapists do not specialise in working directly with the Subconscious, unless they have branched out into hypnotherapy as well. Also, psychology is largely about studying and trying to understand human experience and behaviour - accounting for it, with observations and logical analysis - whereas hypnotherapy is all about changing it, and rapidly too. The psychologist is only really working with the client's *conscious* mind, so if the problem is emotional or habitual, therapy may go on for ages and may never really get anywhere because the conscious mind does not control those things and cannot change them. It is exactly the same with counselling.

Let us consider an example. One of my favourite little tasks as a therapist is clearing flying phobias. Many phobias are easy to get rid of and we usually aim to do it in a single session. In my opinion flying phobias are the easiest of the lot, but of course you have to know how to do it. Without working directly with the Subconscious, removing any serious phobic reaction would be slow and difficult in most cases and impossible in many, so it is not surprising that a psychologist who is not also a hypnotherapist would regard phobias as a persistent problem they might seek to help their client contend with, rather than something they can rapidly eliminate which is the way I regard them.

Recently I was wandering through a bookshop at Manchester airport, waiting for my flight to Cyprus to be called when a little self-help book caught my eye entitled "Flying? No Fear!"

published by Summerdale as part of their 'self help' series. The blurb on the back cover said:

> Written by an airline pilot and a clinical psychologist, this combination of practical explanation and self-help techniques is the definitive guide to help anyone overcome their fear of flying.

Since the book itself is tiny – small enough to fit into the breast-pocket of a shirt – it may not be comforting to the phobic to be told that this modest work is "the definitive guide" to overcoming his condition, but some of it certainly is interesting. I particularly enjoyed reading the reassurances of the airline pilot Captain Adrian Akers-Douglas, whose very name sounds like a type of aircraft. Most of what he writes is actually quite helpful but there are moments in the 'definitive guide' where he reveals a striking lack of appreciation for the subtleties of suggestion. Under the alarming sub-heading *I Can't Get Out* he writes:

> Civil airliners do not carry parachutes: for a start, we cannot open the doors in flight (the air pressure inside the cabin makes this impossible, even if the mechanism was operated) and anyway it is highly unlikely that untrained passengers could make a successful parachute descent even if they had time to put on parachutes in an emergency and could 'bail out'. So although you cannot get out, you are in a very safe 'cocoon' whilst you are on board.
>
> P79, Flying? No Fear! Summersdale, 2002

The phobic would read the above passage thus: No time to put on parachutes in an emergency – no parachutes anyway – no point – even if we could get out – which we can't – passengers would die anyway in the descent – can't get out – no-one can – impossible –

doors cannot be opened - no time, we're all going to die we can't get out we are all going to die trapped inside this cocoon-like coffin...

Yeah, thanks Adrian. No offence, but I hope you're not my pilot on this trip to Cyprus. Does he talk to his passengers like that?

> If you look out of the window you will see we are just passing over the Alps, which means an emergency landing would be impossible if anything went wrong with the plane. As you know we do not carry parachutes, so although we did point out the emergency exits earlier they are of no use to you whatsoever at the moment in any event, so you are effectively trapped. Soon we will be back over the ocean though, in which situation the emergency exits are theoretically useful in the event of a ditching, although to be honest none of us have ever had to test that out in reality. The drinks trolley will be along in a moment, so please refrain from running up and down the aisle screaming: "We're doomed, we're doomed!"

I should be fair: most of what Adrian has to say is interesting and reassuring, logical, rational and sensible. The only trouble is, phobias are not operated by the logical part of the mind. So reassuring the conscious mind is a complete waste of time, as anyone with a serious phobic reaction will tell you. But it is what the Clinical Psychologist - Dr. George Georgiou - has to say that is really ridiculous. Coincidentally it says in the book that he lives and works in Cyprus, the very place I was headed for when I stumbled upon this literary gem.

Dr. Georgiou's expert advice to the phobic reader ranges from various mental coping strategies including positive thinking and basic relaxation techniques, to a detailed explanation of exactly what the phobic experiences should they actually manage to get on the plane. Since the book is ostensibly written for people with a flying phobia, it is inconceivable that those people should need the experience of a phobic reaction describing to them in harrowing detail, but that is what he does. Then there is advice on diet and nutrition, vitamins, herbal remedies and Dr Bach's Rescue Remedy, which many of my phobic clients mention having tried. Clearly it didn't solve their problem or they would not have felt the need to consult me. It is nevertheless described in the book, almost hysterically, as "an absolute must!" That is Dr Georgiou's exclamation mark, not mine.

Hypnotherapy is not mentioned once anywhere in the book. Is that because Dr Georgiou is completely unaware that many people get rid of phobias easily that way? I find that impossible to believe, which would indicate that he is not mentioning hypnotherapy most deliberately. He does, however, find time to include detailed instructions upon how to use a relaxation technique coupled with guided imagery and controlled breathing which does in fact amount to self hypnosis, although he never refers to it as such. In mild cases that might even be quite useful. But in all cases of serious phobic reactions I would regard that approach as being less effective than prayer. Phobics with severe reactions need a cure, but this clinical psychologist seems to think that an outright cure is beyond the bounds of possibility. This is how George Georgiou begins his section:

> I believe that it is very important for anyone who suffers from anxiety or phobias to understand fully what is happening to them during an anxiety attack. Understanding the symptoms is the first step to being able to combat them.

This sums up the whole of the psychological approach: it is all about trying to fight against the reaction with a conscious effort and the application of rationality - as if the reaction is inevitable but you can somehow 'keep a lid on it' by reasoning with yourself. Feel free to emit a hollow laugh if you personally have a strong phobic reaction to any object or situation. One session with Dr Georgiou talking at you like this, and you would probably want to smash him over the head with one of the weighty psychology books with which I'm sure his office is adorned. Don't use the little 'definitive guide' though - he'd hardly feel a thing.

> Gaining a detailed understanding of what is happening to your mind and body during an anxiety attack will facilitate your ability to control the situation. It will also help put into perspective those distorted feelings of impending danger that surface, hence alleviating the intensity of the attack.

Hence doing nothing of the kind, George. There speaks a man who has never had an anxiety attack himself – or not a severe one anyway. Dr. Georgiou writes in detail about all sorts of changes going on in the body as well as the awful experience of the reaction, without once realising that all this is being deliberately orchestrated by the Subconscious mind and that there are real reasons for that, particular to that individual. The Clinical Psychologist clearly does not understand that this can be stopped altogether by an effective therapeutic intervention: it can be shut down completely with hypnotherapy – indeed, I find that really easy to do . Instead, Dr. Georgiou is of the opinion that:

> The person who suffers from anxiety and phobia is indulging in faulty thinking... Apart from faulty thinking, perhaps the most frightening aspect of the panic attack is the loss of control that the individual has always taken for granted. He or she has to struggle to retain or regain voluntary control over focusing, concentration, attention and action. At times, the difficulty in focusing extends to a

> sense that he is losing consciousness, although actual loss of consciousness is rare.

Yes, conscious control of these things is being seriously disrupted... *by the Subconscious.* Notice how the psychologist blames the phobic for all this though? For "indulging in faulty thinking"! How patronising is that?

> The body generally prepares itself for the 'flight or fight' reaction that characterises phobic anxiety states...

To use the word "flight" in this context, apparently without noticing the irony of it indicates an over-serious mind, and not a very quick one either. But the real problem with that statement is the idea that the body *prepares itself,* as if the mind has nothing to do with it. Similarly the assumptions in the previous passage about "loss of control" reveal utter ignorance about the role of the Subconscious mind - as if this battle is simply the conscious mind v. the body. These changes in the body, the emotions involved and the overwhelming impulse to escape or avoid the situation are being purposely directed by the phobic's Subconscious mind out of choice, and only because of a misunderstanding. Their conscious mind may have been told many times why all this is unnecessary or unreasonable but no-one has explained that to the Subconscious, and the Clinical Psychologist here – the supposed expert writing the 'definitive guide' – has no experience of that kind of procedure. In other words, he is no expert.

I don't want to tar all psychologists with the same brush, but the notion that psychology is more respectable or reliable than hypnotherapy just because it falls within the general boundaries of 'the scientific' due to the application of logical analysis leads to this kind of ridiculous situation, where a man who cannot cure your condition is being presented as a worthy expert, yet his prejudices and professional insecurity prevent him from mentioning that hypnotherapy is likely to be a damn sight more use than anything else he suggests. It is just about possible, I suppose, that he really does not know anything about what hypnotherapy can achieve, but that would mean he must be a very narrow reader in the field of behavioural therapies and no more usefully informed about the most effective solution than the man in the street. In which case, who asked *him* to contribute to a "definitive guide" on the subject?

No, it is much more likely that he is doing what many scientific and medical authorities do nowadays, which is exiling hypnotherapy deliberately by omission, literally acting as if it does not exist.

## Hypnotherapists Who Call Themselves Psychologists

It is perhaps understandable then why many psychologists prefer to ignore or rubbish hypnotherapy, since a real acceptance of it would force them to question the usefulness of psychology. But why do some hypnotherapists also offer "psychotherapy" or refer to themselves as psychologists as well as hypnotherapists? Well it is sad to say, but there are probably quite a few professional hypnotherapists out there who suspect they will be more highly regarded by the therapy-seeking public if they also call themselves psychologists, or advertise psychotherapy as well as hypnotherapy. They may hope that it sounds more scientific and therefore more generally acceptable - considerations that are more about profile than methodology. Some of these practitioners may actually have some qualification in psychology, but others don't because let's face it, any talking cure can be loosely regarded as psychotherapy, in that it is about the mind (the psyche), and supposed to be therapeutic.

But what of the others? Why would someone with a genuine, in-depth knowledge of hypnotherapy - who was experienced and confident in its use - bother with psychology? Well, I'm not going to pretend I know for sure and I may be wrong, but my feeling is that therapists in fact either lean more to one side or the other. Either these people are really psychologists who don't have much practical experience of hypnotherapy at all, i.e. they don't actually use hypnosis ordinarily, they just did a course on it once and they like to appear to have more than one string to their bow. The fact that they rarely use it means that they will have little experience and therefore not much confidence in their hypnotherapy skills, but they like to imagine they can do that too. Consequently they may have convinced themselves that hypnotherapy is of limited use when really it is their personal limitations in that area making it appear so. Or they are really hypnotherapists, who had a background in psychology originally then discovered hypnosis and NLP... but they don't think it will do them any harm to mention psychotherapy on their business card.

Can a psychologist become an expert with hypnotherapy too and yet remain a psychologist? If they want to call themselves that, yes. But I would argue that any therapist who uses hypnotherapy regularly and with consistent success is a hypnotherapist. Any therapist who does not use it regularly - and only has modest success if they do - is not a hypnotherapist, but a dabbler. The question is, why would anyone who has become an expert in hypnotherapy still prefer to call themselves a psychologist? Surely it can only be because of the ignorance and prejudice that still affects public perceptions of hypnosis. And it is up to people who genuinely become expert in these matters to change that, because no-one else can.

## Conscious Therapy v. Subconscious Therapy

Here is the real difference between psychology and hypnotherapy. When the psychologist intervenes to help a person with a problem, they are bringing their conscious faculties to bear upon that issue. In other words, they are not only talking to the other person's conscious mind and failing to address that person's Subconscious issues at all, but they are also relying upon their own conscious reasoning alone to fix the problem.

In hypnotherapy, we not only explain matters in detail to the client's conscious mind – that is the function of the pre-talk, and should never be neglected – but we then go on to talk to the client's Subconscious *and that part of the session is conducted by the therapist's Subconscious,* unless of course they are a beginner or a dabbler. Every expert hypnotherapist will be bringing the unlimited creative power of the Imagination to bear upon the problem, generating new creative solutions spontaneously according to that individual's needs, right when they need it.

Real hypnotherapy is live and generally unplanned - there is no pre-planned script where the expert is concerned. It is an imaginative and creative process of communication, not analysis or logical reasoning. In other words it is an art, not a science – and that is why anyone who is more comfortable in the field of the 'mind sciences' like psychology will never feel comfortable with hypnotherapy and is therefore very unlikely to become an expert.

This also means they are also unlikely to become an enthusiastic advocate of hypnotherapy because they are not going to have much personal experience of the dramatic success it can achieve. On the contrary, they are likely to doubt such dramatic and rapid success is possible because it certainly isn't the norm with psychotherapy - and few therapists want to contemplate the possibility that there is a much more successful method available than the one they have spent years learning about. Perhaps it is better to pretend that there isn't, or that such techniques are unproven, or that it is dangerous, or hocus-pocus, or just isn't... *scientific* enough to be taken seriously.

## Who's Afraid of Hypnosis?

Look at the booming and lucrative professional field known as "Sports Psychology". This is a major phenomenon now, but most sports people don't realise it is pretty much all hypnosis and NLP. It's just that you cannot approach big sporting organisations with something called "hypnosis" - you'll scare the poor dears. They will have visions of their centre-forward barking like a dog every time he scores a goal. But if you call it Sports Psychology, that's fine - that's nice and safe and scientific, nobody is afraid of that. The trouble is, 'psychology' then gets the credit for what hypnosis and NLP achieve, and the public go on believing that the only thing you can do with hypnosis is make someone do the funky chicken whenever the music plays.

So I'm standing up for hypnotherapy here. You see, what I do – the wonderful, distinct, and particular art of hypnotherapy - is not psychology, nor is it a branch of psychology. It is not psychoanalysis. It is not analysis of any sort. It is not counselling. It is nothing to do with psychiatry, or the mentally ill. It has nothing whatsoever to do with stage hypnosis. It is not 'mind control by somebody else', or brainwashing. The client's Subconscious mind controls the whole thing - not the hypnotist - and does what it likes with the hypnotist's suggestions, which carry no weight of their own.

Very often hypnotherapy is not about people who have something wrong with them. It is a way for ordinary people to improve their quality of life in a hundred different ways, easily altering or correcting things that the conscious mind has found it cannot alter or correct for the simple reason that it was never in a position to do so. And all this is achieved by relaxing in a comfortable chair for an hour or so while someone else explains the situation to your Subconscious mind, pointing out what changes you want the Subconscious to take care of and why it's a good idea. As the client, you don't even have to *listen* on a conscious level, although you can if you like. It is your Subconscious mind that carries out the adjustments and you don't even notice that happening because it is going on beneath the usual level of consciousness. You are just aware that you are relaxing in a comfortable chair and you feel perfectly normal. You can hear everything as normal, you are not asleep. During this, the client and the therapist can chat, quite ordinarily. Or the client can just relax. It's like dozing in an armchair when you aren't actually asleep, just resting your eyes.

Then afterwards - and much to your conscious mind's astonishment, because it didn't do anything - you find you suddenly have no desire to eat chocolate anymore, or smoke cannabis, or tobacco. You are no longer terrified of frogs. Your weight starts to come down. The panic attacks have gone. You no longer feel sick each time you see him go by in his car, with her. In fact, she's welcome to him, he's a loser! Now you no longer feel like murdering your boss, you are just applying for a better job. Driving test? Exam nerves? Best Man speech? No problem at all. That so-called "intractable" pain from my old knee injury is gone - they told me at the pain clinic I'd have that for the rest of my life. My psoriasis has improved. My asthma is much better. I still carry my inhaler, but so far I haven't needed to use it.

I no longer feel like a loser in the game of life. I hardly drink now, thanks to you! I was worried I was becoming an alcoholic. I thought I must have one of those "addictive personalities", until you explained why that was all nonsense and revealed what was really going on - it's just a compulsive habit! It was never outside my control, just outside my *conscious* control. My Subconscious was controlling it fine, and just didn't know I had made a conscious decision to change that. Now I no longer get cravings to reach for a drink when I get home from work. I just feel indifferent to it, just like I did at 10am. It all makes sense now! Of course I wasn't addicted... how can you be *un*-addicted all day long then suddenly become hopelessly addicted at six o'clock in the evening? Compulsive habit, of course it is. And easy to change - just a little bit of expert hypnotherapy, that's all we need.

Now I'm okay on motorways. I really enjoy riding in aircraft again, just like I did when I was a kid. My acting skills have improved so much now you've got rid of my stage fright. To think, I nearly gave it up! I never thought of hypnotherapy until my hairdresser mentioned you. You helped her mother get through that court-case, remember how anxious she was?

I just had to ring and tell you – I got the job!

No, I am not a victim anymore. I am a survivor, and I actually feel like one now, too. And I'm going to be okay. I have so much more confidence now, after those two sessions.

So come on - what do you think? Ten years with a psychologist? A nine-month waiting-list, followed by twelve sessions of counselling on the NHS and the problem still there at the end? Valium? Beta-blockers? Patches? Zyban? Anti-depressants? Prozac? Seventeen different medications from the GP, half of them to counteract the side-effects of the others?

Or would you rather relax in a comfy chair and find out what the human Subconscious can do? You can be absolutely certain there will be no risk, no side-effects, no loss of control, no equipment, no medication, no willpower needed, no conscious efforts required whatsoever. This is hypnotherapy: and when it is done properly it wipes the floor with any other mental therapeutic intervention in the world – sometimes in just one session - because there is no corrective mechanism more powerful than the human Subconscious mind.

Oh dear. I suppose I've thoroughly alienated any number of readers with a background or profession in the 'mind sciences'. Oh well. Never mind. You can't make an omelette without breaking eggs. The 'mind sciences' have usually been more than happy to slate, alienate and generally ignore hypnotherapists for a century or more, and Dr. Georgiou's not-very-definitive guide, which fails to mention hypnotherapy at all, is a perfect and all-too-common example of that. And that's why it's no good.

# Section Fourteen

## Those Two Imposters: Success and Failure

- ❖ - Success Rates
- ❖ - Relapse is not Failure
- ❖ - Removing the Fear of Failure

*"If you can meet with Triumph and Disaster,
And treat those two imposters just the same..."*

from "If", by Rudyard Kipling

What does Kipling mean when he describes both success and failure as "imposters"? Surely success is success, and failure is failure, right? How can they be anything else?

On the face of it, yes. But Kipling is being more philosophical about each, suggesting a *wiser* way of looking at immediate results - and people can easily understand it too, which is one of the reasons this poem was recently voted the British public's favourite poem of all time. In this section we will be looking at concepts of 'success' and 'failure' and examine how those words function as suggestions, generate trends and influence outcomes. Also how we can turn those things to our advantage, both in therapy and - as Kipling suggests - in life.

"Nothing succeeds like success", as the saying goes – which is a bit like saying: "Nothing is quite as sunny as the sun!" if you look at it literally.

But if we consider these expressions *as suggestions* – for that is how they function, in common usage – then we begin to see how people are inspired, or discouraged, by the suggestions they pick up on and then often repeat to themselves, or those that are directed at them by others. There is no power in a suggestion, it is how you feel about the suggestion that counts - and there can be many factors influencing our feelings when it comes to deciding which suggestion has the most significance for us, and which is meaningless, too good to be true, or just outside our usual experience.

But first we should consider, since we are aiming to achieve it: what is Success? How do we recognise it, how do we measure it, and how will we know when we have actually secured lasting success?

## Success Rates

When people ring me up to ask about my services, a common question is: "What are your success rates?" And it seems a reasonable enough question on the face of it, does is not? Now, just imagine that you are the hypnotherapist, and you have to answer that question. A smoker has contacted you to investigate the possibility of getting rid of his smoking habit, and directly asks you how successful your methods are. What are you going to say?

Well, you might immediately assume that you would simply 'tell the truth'. Absolutely, and very commendable of course, everyone would agree. But the first real problem with that is this: there isn't a therapist in the land who knows what the 'true' answer to that question is. Let me explain what I mean. If a person comes to my office to stop smoking, and stops smoking, that would seem to count as a success. But unless I call them up a month later, how do I know if they are still a success or not? What about six months later? A year? Two years? What if they start smoking again seven years later? Does that turn them, statistically, from a success into a failure? That is the first technical problem with 'success rates' - what actually counts, and what does not count, as a success?

If any incidence of relapse, sooner or later, statistically converts a success into a failure then in order to have an accurate figure for the ongoing rate of success I would have to keep tabs on every one of the hundreds of clients I see for quitting smoking every year. In fact I would have to keep contacting them all regularly, for years on end, to be sure it was still accurate! The cost in terms of time alone, never mind call charges, would make that utterly impossible. Also this would amount to pestering clients in a quite unthinkable way.

Yet even if I could do that, I would not know for sure how accurate any of that was because I would only have that client's word for their success status. Imagine being a smoker who quits initially but later picks up the habit again. If your hypnotherapist suddenly telephones to check your quit-status, you may feel embarrassed to admit that you started again. Or just taken by surprise and not ready to deal with the issue right at that moment. You might be tempted to pretend all was well even if it wasn't, might you not? Of course not everyone would do that, but there are those who tend to just tell people what they want to hear, especially if they are put on the spot. So how accurate are the 'success rates' going to be anyway, if we actually did try to monitor it ourselves that way?

## NHS 'Success'

The NHS Stop Smoking clinics will chalk you up as an official "non-smoker" if you report not smoking for four weeks. This is in line with Department of Health guidelines but as a method of recording real, lasting success it is dubious to say the least!

However, they have the same problem the rest of us have: if you are going to comment on "success" at all, where do you draw the line and how do you analyse the success of your own methods in any meaningful way?

The trouble is, if you start talking about the complexities of measuring success it may begin to sound as if you are trying to create a smoke-screen, as it were, so that you do not have to talk about actual success, as if you have something to hide. But if we do not address the real problems with this, different therapy practices can end up claiming success rates that nobody believes, and that is no use to any of us. Some practitioners within the field of hypnotherapy have been known to claim up to 95% success rates for smoking - and even though I know that is not accurate, I do understand why they do that. There are two reasons:

### 1. We have to Sell Hypnotherapy, as well as provide it

If we wish to assist somebody to achieve any goal, the first thing a hypnotherapist must do is *sell the method* as an ideal route to that outcome. We can only begin to help a client once they are seated before us, so the first challenge is to achieve that. Most people who contact me have never had hypnotherapy before, so they tend to be uncertain about a number of things, and they really need me to demonstrate total confidence in my own abilities and lots of reassurance that they, personally, are going to be successful.

A client told me recently that he had phoned another hypnotherapist asking about weight loss, only to be told it would "take several sessions, and it might work or it might not". Think about it: how would you feel about booking a few sessions with that clown? Hypnotherapists are supposed to be masters of suggestion! "It might work or it might not"? What kind of fool would say that to a client when they first ring up? Needless to say, there was no booking. So there was *no weight loss, guaranteed*. Way to go, hypnotist! You fell at the first fence there, and took the client down with you.

"Hang on though," I hear some of you cry, "Wasn't he just being honest?" Yes he was, and just look how much good that did either of them. There are lots of ways you can be honest without ruining an opportunity for success. Everybody *knows* it might work or it might not, they already have those doubts. So just by *speaking those words* you are reinforcing that doubt quite unnecessarily, and that is a great way to lose a booking and really let your client down. This is not what the client needs to hear. Can you imagine a pharmacist selling you nicotine patches, then just as you head for the door, saying: "By the way, statistically this is pretty unlikely to work"? Literally that is true. Strictly speaking he is being honest but he certainly isn't being *any help*, because now that the pharmacist has said that, you are even less likely to succeed than you were before he opened his stupid fat gob.

Sorry, that was a bit unnecessarily rude. Especially since this is a fictional pharmacist anyway. I'm sure no real pharmacist would be so unnecessarily honest about the poor success rates of NRT. Wouldn't sell many patches then, would they? No.

## 2. We know the Impact of the Initial Suggestion

When the prospective client asks what the success rate is, as a therapist you have to consider *their best interests* in deciding what to tell them. Everything you say will play a significant part in the overall attempt to be successful. After they put the phone down, they will have plenty of time to dwell on what you said to them. If what you said was 100% positive, they can build up their hopes and therefore their *real* chances of success. But if you said something dumb – and we've all done it, at one time or another - they have plenty of time to chew on that before the session comes around, and that *actively diminishes* their expectations and very likely their subsequent *response.*

So, given that you *do not know in advance* any real or accurate answer, if you are going to answer that question about success rates at all, it has to be a fictional answer. And whatever you say, it is going to function entirely as a suggestion, which may well play a major part in their imminent decision on booking a session, *and* their later decision as to whether or not to bother turning up for that session. It may also have a real bearing on their actual response during the session, because it is all suggestion at the end of the day. It all counts, every suggestion plays its part. From the hypnotherapist's point of view, then, he owes it to his client as well as himself to suggest very positive prospects for success, one way or another, as a first stage in creating that success for real.

From this point of view it seems quite logical, then, to claim a very high success rate. Not too high, though - it has to be believable. No-one but a fool would believe a claim to a 100% success-rate, obviously. So: where to pitch that fictional figure? 95%? 90%? 85%? 80%? 75%? 70%? It all becomes meaningless, really, doesn't it? At what point does doubt creep in, for you? Even if you say 95%, some people will immediately assume that *they* are going to be within that 5% "failure" bracket, because whatever they are prepared to believe about the therapist's success, they have zero faith in their own capacity for success.

So although it is understandable that people should ask about "success rates" - and also understandable that hypnotherapists might regard it as entirely in the client's interests to claim very high success rates, as well as their own interests - actually it is an impossible question to answer without the answer causing some sort of problem, whatever success rate you choose to claim. And if something is impossible, what you need is a safe way around it. This isn't just being evasive by the way - this is an intelligent response to a no-win situation.

What do I tell my prospective clients these days, when they ask what my success rates are? I simply advise them that we are not allowed to quote figures at them - it is against advertising law to do that, even over the phone. (I have no idea exactly how true that is, by the way, and I don't care, because I am not doing it anyway.) I then add that I think this restriction is quite right, as it prevents anyone making ridiculous claims – a point they naturally agree with. This agreement unites the client and me in our mutual disapproval of OTHER therapists making false claims. Not that they necessarily are of course - but that is not certain, whereas it is plainly evident that I am not. I then assure my prospective client with great confidence that I know what I'm doing (which is entirely true, *and* exactly what they need to hear)... and that all I really need from them is a genuine preference to be a non-smoker, which they always assure me that they have. (Of course they have, that's why they rang me.) I have been honest, they are reassured, and I don't have to pluck imaginary figures from the air – ideal solution, really.

Except – ah yes, some of you are still wondering what my 'real' success rates are, aren't you? Well, I'll tell you. I am always successful, in the sense that however the client chooses to respond I get paid anyway and the majority of my clients recommend my services with enthusiasm, which is the best any real practitioner can hope for. What you are really wondering about is exactly how many of my clients are successful, isn't that more precise? And since success in hypnotherapy is directly caused, not by the suggestions I utter, but by the client's Subconscious response to those suggestions, when they do respond successfully that is *their success,* not mine. I have no right to lay claim to that success because I didn't do it, they did. And if they *don't* do it, there isn't a damn thing I can do about it, so it isn't any failure of mine. As long as I did everything necessary, for my part, then I am comfortable with the fact that most people will respond wonderfully well, and a few people will not. Yes, I'm quite comfortable with the knowledge and the expectation that some people will hang on to their problem because the truth is, however expert any hypnotherapist is, some people will.

Is that failure? Only if you (or they) interpret that situation in those terms. To me, there is only success... whether we have arrived at it yet or not. What some people would call a 'failure' I would simply call a person who has not yet achieved their goal. There is a difference - the word 'failure' does not truly describe a reality as many would assume, but is a negative assumption that actively discourages new attempts to succeed and almost rules out the hope of success altogether because it is such a dispiriting notion.

"If at first you don't succeed," the saying goes, "try, try and try again." This is a slightly more hopeful suggestion, because it doesn't mention failure directly. But it does actually imply multiple failures, as if we should assume the next attempt isn't going to work either, and at no point does it promise any actual success. Also, it sounds like very hard work, so it is not appealing at all. If we are going to give ourselves suggestions – and *we are*, whether we recognise them as such or not - we should at least make them promising and appealing. Readily acceptable, comfortable and memorable, inspirational, uplifting and energising.

How about this suggestion:

> "You cannot prevent success, you can only delay it!"

For example: a pole-vaulter from Warrington wishes to smash the world-record for pole-vaulting and establish himself as the most successful pole-vaulter in the world (why does anyone bother?) but the Yemeni reigning champion is determined to stop him, so the night before the competition he sneaks a hungry tiger into the challenger's Winnebago and the challenger loses the ensuing mauling competition which he never would have entered had there been an option b). The next morning's gruesome news has the reigning champion rubbing his hands with glee ("he always kept a tin handy" – Spike Milligan) but not for long – the record is smashed anyway by the Jamaican contender! Yes, I know – who would have thought a Jamaican could get higher than anyone else? Later the killing is linked to the Yemeni when a feeding bowl full of Frosties is discovered along with tiger hair in the back of his Toyota Land Cruiser. At his trial he admitted all, and warned:

"You cannot prevent success, you can only delay it!"

Though he was referring to the success of others, this principle can equally be applied to your own. The suggestion leaves open the obvious factual possibility that you could, if you were really determined to, delay it indefinitely - but at the same time that is not your only option. It also indicates that you are actually controlling the whole thing and the moment you decide to stop delaying success it will come much more easily, which is quite true. Many people are actively delaying their own success - by pursuing the wrong course, by drinking too much, gambling, putting themselves down, keeping the wrong company, denying realities, whatever.

There is a saying in NLP of which I am particularly fond: "If you go on doing the same thing, you'll get the same results." At some point in life, many of us realise this and do something about it, i.e. we stop delaying success. "You cannot prevent success, you can only delay it!" makes the eventual successful outcome seem almost inevitable and any continued attempts to delay it further then appear futile, undesirable and frankly just too much of an effort in the end.

You see, it's all down to how we are talking to ourselves, and each other. A woman once said to me with a heavy sigh: "I just *know* I'm never going to pass my driving test!" Well, no – not as long as you are talking to yourself like that. But if you just change the script: "I don't care what it takes - I'm going to get that licence!" That creates a different mood altogether and naturally a different outcome.

Likewise if someone breezes into a hypnotherapy session with this attitude: "I don't care how many sessions it takes, this problem is history!"...guess how many sessions are likely to be required? That's right, one. But if they start out by asking me:

> "What if it doesn't work? Because I don't want to waste my money on something that doesn't work. What guarantee can you give me that I won't still be smoking after the session?"

...that person is focusing on failure to the exclusion of everything else, and we would have to change that negative dynamic if we are going to create success. I can help them to do that.

## Relapse is Not Failure

Sometimes an ex-smoker will call me up at a later date to report a problem. How they actually report it, the words they feel inclined to use, tells me a lot about the attitude they have decided to take towards this development, and this will be the emotional starting-point for session two.

Now that I have dealt with the issue of success rates, you will already know that all reported figures about outcomes should be regarded as some sort of rough working estimate, and that in the case of smoking particularly, very high figures like 95% should be regarded as promotional. My estimate for my own outcomes, on average, would be about the same as the one made in 1992 by Christopher Pattinson, academic chairman of the British Society of Medical and Dental Hypnosis, as reported in *New Scientist*. He said modern hypnotherapy techniques can be expected to achieve 60% success rates from a single session, and what this means in practice is that sometime after that first session, 40% will need a back-up session at some point.

Some need it straight away, because there is a conflict or stumbling block preventing immediate response, as in some of the Case Mysteries, which I hope have been enlightening regarding such things. Some relapse a few weeks or months later, either just through ordinary carelessness, or some upheaval in their life. Then again, some don't smoke at all for years, and then pick it up again later for no significant reason – rather like the way most of us started smoking tobacco in the first place, in fact.

## Hypnotherapy does not "wear off"!

This is somthing I wanted to be very clear about, because it is one of those notions that really irritate hypnotherapists but are common misunderstandings, rather like the idea of being 'out of control' whilst in hypnosis. It is nonsense, but it is very commonplace nonsense.

Can you imagine somebody saying: "I only started smoking because all my friends were doing it, it was their influence really, but later *the effects of that wore off,* and I stopped." Nobody would dream of saying such a thing, they would never put it like that. Yet we do sometimes hear this: "I stopped smoking with hypnotherapy, but later *the effects wore off* and I started again."

Partly this misunderstanding comes from stage hypnosis, where temporary immediate effects are the norm because that is just a show. Permanent effects would be completely inappropriate, and obviously the stage hypnotist is not aiming to create any permanent changes at all. But this skeptical conscious assumption – that hypnotherapy is some sort of artificial effect that must surely 'wear off' at some stage - also amounts to a commonplace *conscious dismissal* of hypnotherapy. The conscious mind prefers a notion of hypnotherapy as 'temporary' and 'hit-and-miss', because it can scarcely accept the effortlessness of hypnotherapy as a reality in the first place, it sounds too good to be true. Thirdly, the conscious mind sometimes has petty resentment toward the Subconscious, a kind of mental sibling rivalry because it had previously been flattered to believe in its own supremacy, and now it is being suggested that the Subconscious can easily do things the conscious mind has consistently failed to achieve? The conscious mind is competitive, so in a way it does not *want* the Subconscious to turn out to be that effective, as it would seem to diminish its own 'primary' status. This is one reason why some friends or colleagues can be openly gleeful if your hypnotherapy progress encounters delayed success, or relapse. If it is totally successful their skeptical assumptions are proved wrong, which is less welcome than being proved right.

Some readers may find the idea of an active rivalry between the conscious mind and the Subconscious far-fetched but in practice they are often in conflict to some degree. The "resentment" I mentioned seems largely on the conscious side though, and it is useful to bear in mind that this is mostly the effect of educational methods which mislead the conscious mind into believing it directs all decisions and behaviour. The later resentment is a reaction to the effective demotion of the conscious mind upon realising the error in this. Denial is also a common reaction, simply declaring that hypnosis is "all a load of rubbish". It takes zero mental effort to process that piece of mental excrement.

The fourth factor in play, in this notion of hypnotherapy "wearing off", is the idea of hypnotherapy as a *treatment*. Unfortunately, my profession is regarded as "alternative medicine", and so sessions are regarded as treatment. In the sentence:

> "I stopped smoking with hypnotherapy, but later *the effects wore off* and I started again."

...smoking is being regarded as 'the norm', hypnotherapy as 'the treatment being applied', and then the norm being re-established as that 'dose' of hypnotherapy 'wore off'. Most people probably think of hypnotherapy in these terms, whether they realise it or not. So when the smokers from the 40% who will need further help at some stage call me back, sometime after session one, they may report the development in that way. Or indeed in various other possible ways:

"It's worn off. Tell me, is it going to wear off every time, like this? Because I can't afford to keep coming back to see you every six months!"

"It's not worked!"

"I'm struggling, I need some help!"

"I don't understand it. I was fine for a month. Then I went on holiday..."

"I was absolutely fine, for two years - never wanted one – I was telling everyone about you, and all about hypnotherapy! Then I found out my husband was having an affair with my sister..."

"I've fallen off the wagon. I am SO annoyed with myself – I was doing so well!"

"I need to come back, I've been smoking in secret for three months now, it's just becoming ridiculous..."

"I'm afraid you're going to be really cross with me... I've started smoking again..."

"Please don't shout at me, but..."

Actually, I don't care. It is none of my business whether you smoke or not. Obviously we aim to succeed immediately, because that is a win-win situation. But I've been doing this for years now, and I have worked with thousands of smokers. Do you honestly think I have any personal feelings about whether any particular client turns out to be one of the 60% who need no further help, or one of the 40% who will? All of these are everyday outcomes to me. But some people imagine I do care, because they've got the whole thing wrong in their heads - misunderstanding who I am and what I do. Some of that 40% who need further help *never ring me back at all* because they are embarrassed or afraid I will be disappointed or upset, feel the same way they do about it or think badly of them.

Listen: when a surgeon contemplates the cases lined up for him or her that week, they know that most of them are going to be well on the road to recovery by the end of the week. They don't know which ones. But they also know, for sure, that a certain proportion of them are not going to be, because they may need more surgery at some point for some reason. There is a fair chance that one or two of the more critical cases will get no further down the road to recovery this time around, because they stall on the level crossing of fate, and the speeding express train of doom - which is a sleeper, of course – will plough into the fragile vehicle of their present incarnation and they will be hurled...

Isn't it curious when a seemingly innocent metaphor gets completely out of hand like that? We started with the 'road to recovery', and just look at what my Subconscious did with that - just for fun! All I was really going to say was, you could not *be* a surgeon, or a therapist, if you had not come to terms with this everyday reality. The surgeon cannot save and heal people without courage, which means outcomes must not be feared. It takes a special kind of person, then, to become an expert in surgery because it is essential to able to live with *all your outcomes,* not just your successes, which anyone could live with, let's face it.

The same principle is true for the hypnotherapist, except it is much easier for us. There is nothing to fear because the worst of all possible outcomes is that nothing happens. I'm not doing cartwheels all the way home when that happens, but neither am I curled up in the corner, sobbing "I'm no good! That poor woman is *still* suffering from feelings of insane jealousy, and it's all my fault!" ...because I know it is not my fault.

Now, that does not mean it is *her* fault, either. That would be a misunderstanding, and a negative judgement, and hypnotherapy does not recognise any kind of usefulness in misunderstandings or negative judgements. In terms of outcomes, for hypnotherapy there can only be:

1. Things that will change immediately and never need further session time spent on that. An A.1 response.
2. Things that change immediately, but need further session time in due course – whether that is soon after, or much later. An A.2 response.
3. Things that don't change immediately, but change after further session time, and remain fine after that. An A.3 response.
4. Things that don't change immediately, but change after further session time, and turn out to need further session time still later on. A.4
5. Things that don't respond to sessions 1 or 2, but do respond to 3, and are fine after that because we located and cleared the thing that stalled sessions 1 and 2. A.5

Just continue in that vein. Notice how *everything* is classed as an 'A' response, because there are no 'inferior' responses. This is a process, not a magic trick. Success is success whenever it happens to occur, and each case is different. If someone does not stop smoking after the first session, they have *not failed,* even if they assume they have. They can certainly turn that *into* a failure, by not calling me back and proceeding no further. A few people do this, but only because they misunderstood what happened.

## The Complaints Procedure

Some people do call me, but don't book another session because they really only called me to complain. This is inappropriate, because I tell all smokers at the end of session one:

> What we expect is total success, so if you have any difficulty later on, simply call me, because I would know exactly what to do about that should it occur.

This clearly indicates we would need to *do something* about it. What I did *not* say is:

> What we expect is total success. If you have any difficulty later on, simply complain. Who knows, you might be able to get your money back even though you obviously haven't really been listening to my detailed explanations of how hypnotherapy really works and how to respond to it, which is one reason your response is delayed anyway.

What do *you* think? Having engaged my services and paid me for my professional time on just one occasion, does anyone deserve a refund for ignoring my advice about how to deal with delays and abandoning an attempt to succeed at the first sign of a hitch?

## Success that happened to be delayed a bit

Some do book a further session but cancel it later, or simply do not turn up. Of the smokers that book a second session and actually turn up, about 75% of those will be successful at that point, because the second session I do on smoking is very effective at eliminating hesitancy when linked with the first. These two sessions are quite different, and session two would certainly not have that sort of success by itself. In fact, the second session wouldn't really make a lot of sense to a person who had never had the first session. It is important to go about these things in a methodical way.

Even then, there will be a few for whom success is yet delayed. Everyone can handle immediate success of course, but how do people handle *delayed* success? Different people will lose heart at different points in the process, and convert this delay into real failure. This may depend upon a number of things: how motivated they are to achieve that particular goal anyway, how much money they have available for therapy at the time, how they react to success that is not immediate, and how they adjust to that, their intellectual understanding of the process (it is a *learning* process, after all – some people never really get that, they keep waiting for me to *fix them*). What advice they are getting from people around them. Whether they are prepared to tackle a particular emotional complication...

Is this failure? Not to me, but it depends what the client decides it is, and at what point they decide this. And of course, we all know that there will be a few people who are simply not going to stop smoking at that point in their lives no matter what anyone does, and every smoker is wondering if that is the case for them, or whether it is worth booking another session. Maybe I am just trying to make as much money as I can out of them, eh?

They have to consider that possibility too.

So I make it easy for them. If someone has not stopped after session 2, and I honestly have no idea why, then I simply explain that I do not recommend a third session with myself at that point. Now, some people are not put off by that, because they have decided they are going to stop, and they have decided to stick with me because everything I have said so far made sense to them, or I had previously helped someone they know. So if they are determined to proceed, I am happy to do so because there is nothing wrong with that attitude and all we need to do is locate the hitch. But if the client seems to be less sure about myself at that point – which is perfectly understandable - I will recommend that they either leave it for a little while and then try again, or try another therapist. As I have said elsewhere, no therapist is right for everyone.

By giving people options, and not trying to talk them *into* further sessions, it becomes obvious I am not just after the client's money, and that is an important thing for people to know.

I will certainly sell them session two if I can, because nobody should be doubtful about developments at that point - I am doing them a favour, it has a high success rate and needing a second session is normal for some people. For the few people not enjoying success yet after that, we need to look at the thing from all angles, and a hard sell would be inappropriate at that stage, for it would raise suspicion in the mind of any normal person at that point anyway. So if people choose to walk away at that stage, I simply wish them well. In my experience those people would not turn up for a third session anyway if they felt I had pushed them in that direction, so there is no point encouraging them to book it.

Upon abandoning their attempt, such clients may then choose to think that they failed to respond to hypnotherapy, or that hypnotherapy failed to 'work' on them. My understanding of that scenario is that they just stopped using hypnotherapy when they did not get immediate or rapid success, because they wanted quick success and assumed that anything that is not quick success must be failure.

Now think of all the great things mankind has achieved over the centuries. How many of them would have been achieved with that attitude? Think of your own greatest achievements. Did you approach them like that? Probably not, but that is exactly how most people approach hypnotherapy. Why? Because they have seen stage hypnosis, of course. Yet we get great success in hypnotherapy even so. Just think what kind of success we could be getting with all sorts of issues if people really understood it, and didn't overreact to ordinary delays, didn't keep walking away when really we have really only just started?

## Ordinary Stumbling Blocks

When people 'relapse', that is not a 'failure' any more than being part of the 40% who need further help after session one would be. Whether that relapse happens two weeks later, or twenty-five years later as in one case I dealt with, it is still an ordinary occurrence. It is easy for your Subconscious to amend it too. But clearly something caused that relapse, and we need to locate the cause and clear it, then get the change re-established. It really is as simple as that.

All sorts of factors can trigger a return to smoking, and I'm not going to list them all here because they are fairly common knowledge anyway, but I want to make a clear distinction between two separate things: the *fact* of starting to smoke again, and how the client *chooses to feel* about that fact.

## The Fact of Smoking and the Fact of Not Smoking

This is not a grey area for anyone who has ever had a compulsive smoking habit. There are a few smokers around who have never developed a *habit,* they smoke sporadically and there is not enough of a pattern for the Subconscious to pick up on, in order to run it on autopilot so they remain in conscious control of the behaviour. These people love to annoy habitual smokers with their apparently superhuman ability to 'take it or leave it', this supposedly highly-addictive thing. And habitual smokers are often in awe of this apparent self-control and envy those amazing people, who can actually be a bit smug about the fact that their smoking is occasional. Of course in reality there is nothing impressive about it at all. We all started out doing that, it is just that most smokers accidentally developed a habit later by doing it regularly. These occasional or 'social' smokers were really just being a bit lame about their smoking behaviour, more hesitant and indecisive about the whole business. They didn't commit to it properly. I don't see why that merits admiration!

After having stopped smoking with hypnotherapy, a small proportion of ex-smokers begin to notice one or two of these 'smugees' (that's a better name for them, don't you think?), and somewhere deep down remember a time when they could do that, too. They then begin to imagine that now they once again have 'control' because they are not smoking, perhaps they could get away with just having the odd one, like the occasional smoker. So they try that.

Now, during the Stop Smoking therapy we asked the Subconscious to please shut the smoking behavioural programme down. It was happy to do that, but the brain never intends to learn anything twice. It has already learned all the smoking behaviour-patterns and the social situations, the triggers and signals involved. It is quite happy to shut the whole thing down forever and a day, but what inevitably happens if that person later puts a cigarette – or a cigar, a joint, anything like that – into their mouth again, the brain just assumes: "Oh! We're doing that again, are we?" ...and re-activates the whole smoking programme, *cravings and all*. It is called shooting yourself through the foot.

Some smokers feel immediately, instinctively that this is what they have done. And some don't, because relapse unfolds differently in each case. In reality it makes no practical difference because once any smoking activity has taken place, for the former habitual smoker *full subsequent relapse is assured in virtually all cases.* It is just a matter of time before the smoker recognises that fact. At first, it may seem as if they have got away with it because in some cases there is no immediate urge to smoke again, but sometime after that another urge to smoke will come. Then another, and another. But it might be weeks before the frequency of urges is causing the smoker real concern. During that time it might be easy for them to convince themselves that they still have this thing under control, and that they are not going to go back to smoking full-time, as it were.

But this is just the conscious mind whistling in the dark - conscious intentions have nothing to do with it. Think of it like a boulder at the top of a hill, with a small rock in front of it. That first post-hypnotherapy puff on a cigarette seems like such a small thing, doesn't it? A bit like idly picking up a small rock out of mere curiosity, what harm could it possibly do? As you wander away, you wouldn't notice the boulder wobble. Even as it gradually starts to roll, ever so slowly, nothing dramatic seems to be happening at all. It is only later, as it crashes into the farmhouse at the bottom of the hill at full speed, killing the farmer's wife, his dog and his favourite pig that the smoker thinks: "Ah. Ooops! Now why did I have to go and do a thing like that?"

Exceptions to this scenario – in which the rock just wobbles and then stays where it is - are so rare that they roughly equate to the number of Popes converting to Judaism whilst in office, so it is important smokers are warned in advance. Not everyone heeds the warning, which is why it is also important to make it clear that returning to hypnotherapy to halt the progress of the boulder – preferably *before* it causes some terrible damage – is a much better strategy than whistling and trying to pretend everything is fine.

## Removing the Fear of Failure

This is not a self-help book, although it might prove to be a very helpful book to some people for all sorts of reasons. That can be true of many books, whether they are meant to be self-help books or not. Very often the information in self-help books is useful enough, but how much the process of reading it will actually change your life may depend upon which side of the mind it is aimed at, and whether that part of the mind *responded* to the message of the book, or received the message at all.

To achieve easy and meaningful change regarding any habitual or emotional issue, and also where healing of the body is required, it is essential for the Subconscious to receive the message clearly and unambiguously, and for that part of the mind to be motivated to respond wholeheartedly, as it were. In my view it also helps if the conscious mind is fully informed and understanding it all, so there is maximum harmony of purpose across all mental faculties. Reading alone is unlikely to achieve all this, and in some people the reading process will fall well short of creating that optimum formula for change. The writers of many self-help books are unlikely to know this.

Let me be clear: I am not suggesting that there is anything wrong with that kind of book. All aspirations to improve ourselves and our quality of life are to be welcomed. It is just that the power of that message is dramatically increased if it is received and fully appreciated by both sides of the mind, and the reading process in itself will not do that consistently enough, and in analytical readers, not at all.

Trance is the key factor here. Sometimes when we are reading the conscious mind is dealing with the information and the Subconscious is ignoring it, so we are not in trance. This is always the case when we are reading analytically, for example following the instructions to build flat-pack furniture. The Subconscious has no interest in this, and even the conscious mind is less than enthralled, it just recognises that the instructions are the only clue to assembly so we had better force ourselves to analyse them. This is not a trance state, so the Subconscious is broadly aware of what is happening but is paying virtually no attention to the details of this rather dull matter, it has delegated that task to the part of the mind best equipped to handle it.

Other types of text would be similarly delegated to the conscious mind quite happily, because they really relate to the affairs of the conscious mind anyway: accountancy, law, health and safety regulations, banking, mortgages and investments. These are the sort of subjects the Subconscious has no interest in because they relate to the outside world and material concerns of a practical, rational nature. They are creations of the conscious intellect, ways of organising multiple interests in a civilised society. So if you are reading a mortgage offer, your conscious mind may have some stake in what it says on that document but your Subconscious couldn't care less.

It is the same when programmes covering these matters are broadcast by radio or on television, it is almost impossible for the Subconscious to pay attention long enough to take in details about interest rates or what happened today on Wall Street –

unless of course it is earth-shattering and signals some genuine threat, which is hardly ever the case. I should emphasize here that I am talking about people who do not normally have a particular daily involvement in these matters. It is different for the person whose pulse-rate rises and falls according to movements on the Dow Jones index because they have become closely attuned to it due to an ongoing professional interest which has engaged them on an emotional level too. But for most of us, there is little or no Subconscious stake in such things.

This state of affairs will usually be quite different if the programme or book relates to matters that relate to Subconscious aims and concerns. Pleasures, especially sexual or gastronomic are very likely to catch the Subconscious mind's attention. Thrill-seeking matters, for some: danger, drama, scary or spooky subjects all connect instantly to the Imagination in the Subconscious mind, in a way that a political pamphlet (for example) is very unlikely to do, especially at this point in history. Anything about death or disease can also have us riveted, especially if it might relate to ourselves, we go into trance whilst reading it. We are engrossed – fascinated - we do not wish to be disturbed whilst we take it all in, and if someone takes it from us or distracts us we may become angry or upset. Our emotions have become engaged.

So we may often be reading analytically, with a critical or philosophical mental attitude engaging only conscious processes, in which case none of this information is reaching the Subconscious. I suspect self-help books are often read this way, and one of the problems with that is that conscious memory (a.k.a. short-term memory) is not able to retain much of that for long - even if we find value in what we are reading, it will soon be forgotten. When we read analytically, even if the subject matter relates to our emotions, our bodies or our habitual behaviour this fact may be missed by the Subconscious. There is nothing much the conscious mind can do about those things anyway because it doesn't control those things, so the message is not acted upon by either part of the mind. The result then is little or no change, although the person might still recommend the book because the message made perfect sense to the logical part of the mind that actually read it. It would have made perfect sense to the Subconscious mind too in all probability, but the Subconscious never processed any details, it was just vaguely aware you were reading a book.

Now think of the scariest book you ever read. The most moving film you ever saw. The funniest performance you ever witnessed. The most stunning breaking-news report you ever tuned in to... your Subconscious was paying attention to those messages alright, and you will remember them for the rest of your life. Do you recall the feeling? That's the difference trance makes... and notice that it has nothing to do with relaxation whatsoever. Trance is when you are paying attention with the whole of your being - not just your conscious intellect - and the full power of the mind is brought to bear upon the subject-matter. You take it to heart, and it stays with you.

## What has all this to do with the Fear of Failure?

I was coming to that. Did you think I had gone off at a tangent? There aren't any tangents. This is not a self-help book, therefore when I *explain* about removing the fear of failure - here in these pages – that is not the same as what happens when I explain the same matters to someone while they are in trance. Explanations are usually read analytically, which means that your Subconscious may not be picking up any of this at all. So even if you find the explanation logical and your conscious mind – which is under the impression that *it is the mind,* and so assumes that it controls all your behaviour and choices, or at least *ought to be able to* – thinks the explanation sounds perfectly plausible, and so resolves to remember it in future and live by that from now on, **nevertheless nothing will change**. Committed to short-term memory only, your conscious mind will not remember it for more than a day or two at best - and if the information concerns physical health, emotional or habitual matters, will not be able to change that anyway however much sense it would make on a logical level of conscious processing. Your Subconscious, which can change any of those things without effort or delay anytime you like, never processed the explanation at all. And that is why many self-help books are misconceived – not in the content, but the form.

## Recorded Sound as 'Hypnotherapy'

Some hypnosis books try to get around this by including a CD with a relaxation approach in order to hopefully present the message to the Subconscious as well. This would be a great idea, except for three things:

a. Many readers will not get around to listening to it, or only listen to it *once*, assuming that they then 'know' it
b. if the listener has a significant fear of failure – quite a lot of smokers do - that will tend to dominate their listening experience and so probably scupper any real, wholehearted response, and
c. I have yet to hear any relaxation/suggestion CD that informs the listener *how to respond* to the suggestions on the recording. How are they listening to this CD? With desperation? With doubt? With vague hope, tempered with realism? Are they lying there on the bed thinking: "Well I feel quite relaxed, but I really don't see what difference this is supposed to make! I mean he's just repeating what he said in the book, and that didn't make me any thinner!"

These are lame, worthless attitudes resulting in no change, and this is not the fault of the listener if they have not been given enough information to avoid this. Are they *waiting to see* what the results are? Wondering? Hoping? No good! Or are they responding to the message with enthusiasm, which would be the right attitude to adopt? Not if their fear of failure is blocking it. And anyway, if they haven't been instructed to respond with enthusiasm, how on earth would they know that they should?

## Clearing the Fear of Failure

This is one of the Five Golden Keys of Successful Hypnotherapy, and it did occur to me that maybe I shouldn't tell you what any of them are... that perhaps I should not reveal the Secrets, but reserve them for my most earnest disciples who would first have to prove themselves worthy by a series of gruelling tasks that would defeat most ordinary mortals. Long ago I learned that only True Grandmasters of Suggestion should hold all Five Keys, for their power is awesome. Many days I spent alone, agonising with my soul as to whether I should reveal the secret of this, one of the Very Golden Keys of which I speak. Also, I figured I could probably design a training course called Learn the Secrets of the Five Golden Keys of Successful Hypnotherapy and then charge ridiculous amounts of money for places on the course which only really teaches you things you could learn in an afternoon in any decent library. Yes, do beware of expensive training courses that ruthlessly exploit your self-doubt. As a general rule of thumb: the more expensive they are, the more suspicious you should be.

Okay, it's simple. The reason we should have no fear of failure is because failure does not exist. That's right: there is no such thing as failure. And I know immediately that many readers will react instinctively against that statement thus: "You are simply wrong, fool hypnotist. Everyone knows what failure is, it is an attempt which does not succeed."

Bear with me! I know what people *mean* by the word 'failure', I understand what their concept of it is. It's just that I don't believe it exists in reality. I also know what people mean by the word 'dragon'. I understand their concept of that, too - it's just that I don't believe dragons exist in reality. And even though dragons are traditionally huge, fire-breathing monsters that can fly, the fact that I don't believe they really exist completely saves me from any fear of dragons, as I'm sure you can easily appreciate. So the fact that I do not believe failure exists completely saves me from any fear of failure... and I'm sure you can imagine just how useful that is. So allow me to share it with you.

There is no such thing as failure. There is only success, and delayed success. If you look at the life of any successful person – and you could pick anyone you like from history, a figure that everyone would regard as a success in what they set out to achieve – if you read their biography, I guarantee you will find that their life was not just a success story. No, it will turn out to have been full of obstacles, setbacks, delays and frustrations, as human lives usually are. But what made that person a success in what they set out to do is that they never regarded any of those things as a failure. They regarded them as obstacles, setbacks and delays, and they ploughed on.

There is only success, and delayed success. And of course it is wonderful when you knock on the door of opportunity, and it just swings open immediately - when success just drops into your lap first time of asking. But experience teaches us that this is not usually the way it happens. More likely we will have to knock on many doors, or try various approaches, before we find the thing that works, and by this process finally achieve success. And when success does not just drop into your lap – when you have to work for it, be persistent and determined – then when success does come at last, does it not seem all the more worthwhile for that? Because then you feel you have really earned it, so you deserve it all the more. But either way it is still success, whether it was delayed or not. And no matter how long success is delayed, it is still success.

Hence you are always on the road to success. It is a good road to be on. Every footstep on the road to success brings you closer to your goals. And so you can enjoy every step. You don't have to wait until you reach your goal before you can be happy. Too many people defer happiness, by suggesting to themselves, "I'll be happy when I've got my degree", or "I'll be happy when I've paid off my mortgage". Why not be happy now? Why wait? Then when you get your degree, you can be even happier! Every achievement, every little milestone along the Road to Success creates more happiness and fulfilment, so you just continue... happy to be on The Road to Success, and enjoying it every step of the way.

And when you reach an obstacle you need not be dismayed, or any less happy. Why are people surprised by obstacles? Did they seriously expect there to be none? We should expect them, what great achievement did not involve overcoming obstacles along the way? If we confidently expect obstacles to present themselves from time to time, then they no longer seem such a nasty surprise but become a normal part of what we were expecting all along. For an obstacle is only a temporary problem to a human being. Humans are clever, resourceful and certainly up to the challenge obstacles present. We can find a way around it. We can climb over it, tunnel underneath it, or blast straight through it if that is the way we feel like dealing with it. If you need to inspire yourself with thousands of examples of obstacles being overcome brilliantly, just study human history. And if you wish to broaden the perspective, investigate the natural world – of which we are of course a part.

As for a setback, since when did humans begin to be discouraged by such a trifling occurrence? It is just a setback, we reorganise our plans and expectations accordingly, adjust to the new reality and continue. Look at human endeavours throughout the centuries, there are numerous setbacks everywhere you look - but nothing would be worth achieving if it did not involve such things. Humans are not discouraged easily. And delays? Well, we can be patient. We can be persistent and determined. Delayed success is still success, no matter how long it is delayed.

In fact, the only way you can *create the illusion of failure* is to reach an obstacle or an ordinary setback, sit down, give up and suggest to yourself that you have failed, immediately then accepting that negative suggestion. That is the only way you can do it, and of course that is easy enough to do. In fact any fool can do that, and I suppose we all have done exactly that at one time or another. But we did not have to, and if you never do that, you can never fail. Thus you are always on the road to success if you choose to look at it in that way and reject the negative view, which was no fun anyway. Happy to be on the Road to Success, enjoying every step and looking forward to the successes and the challenges ahead. Let other people believe in a thing called failure, if they think that will help them. Of course it won't, it will haunt them. But for you, the whole notion of failure is about as scary as a dragon. A pink one. A small, fluffy pink dragon with a sticky-out tongue made of fuzzy felt.

Now, notice how you *feel* having read that. If you feel inspired, moved, elated or some similar positive reaction, you dropped into trance at some point and your Subconscious found that point of view appealing. Read it over again, read it a few times and eliminate your fear of failure. Read it at regular intervals in your life. Frame it, put it on the wall or stick it on the fridge perhaps. Only please, don't put it in the downstairs toilet - that really is no place for anything deep and meaningful. It's just not the right setting for an epiphany.

If on the other hand you felt nothing whilst discovering that failure is a mythical concept – if it did not move you at all - either your Subconscious didn't take it in, or else it had no motivation to respond positively. If you *think* it sounded fairly reasonable, but you *feel* no different, then you read it analytically and any fear of failure you may have would not be changed today. But that only means your Subconscious wasn't paying attention, it does not mean the suggestions are no use to you. Also, when I present these thoughts to someone's Subconscious mind in therapy, I put some power and enthusiasm into it. The voice is a powerful tool when it is used appropriately, and can move people far more than ink on a page.

Another thing that can affect the response is how relevant such a message seems to that person at the point in their life when they encounter it. I'm sure Robert the Bruce has seen many spiders rebuilding webs before he witnessed the one that inspired him. As he gazed at the creature determinedly working away with a complete absence of discouragement or depression, he went into a trance and his Imagination created a self-suggestion that lifted his own spirit, and he resolved to re-double his efforts and battle on with renewed energy and zest.

We only need to get the message right, the delivery of the message right and the response right, and we have success. Always. Nobody is excluded. When success is delayed, there is always a reason. But failure it is not. So - it can stay with you forever now. Close your eyes and create a powerful association that will always make you smile and sometimes even save the day:

    failure = fluffy pink dragon

# Section Fifteen

## The Art of Hypnotherapy in Practice

- ❖ - Waking Suggestion
- ❖ - Some Useful Laws of Hypnotherapy
- ❖ - How to Choose a Good Hypnotherapist
- ❖ - How to Accept Suggestions Successfully

## Waking Suggestion

'Waking Suggestion' is a technical term in hypnotherapy for suggestion that is presented when the client is apparently not in trance, or not in trance at all. Actually it is a silly term, since trance has nothing to do with sleep anyway, but then hypnosis is full of terminology that turns out to be misleading once you really understand the workings of it. This is because the terms often originate from earlier phases in the development of the knowledge when it was largely being misunderstood by the pioneers investigating the subject. I would say it is still misunderstood in some ways even by successful hypnotists, which is why I would not expect all of them to agree with everything I state in this book.

I believe that the most *successful* therapists of any sort, whether they formally use 'hypnosis' or not, have really become skilled in the presentation of waking suggestion – as are the most successful salespeople, advertisers and promoters of all types. (At one time we could probably have said the same about successful politicians, but nowadays their main communication skill seems to be evasion.)

The general popular assumption about hypnotherapy – the idea that we 'put' people in a trance and then simply tell them what to do, as in: "From now on, you will hate the smell of cigarettes!" - is really just a face-value assumption about *stage* hypnosis, transposed onto the therapy scenario. Unfortunately, I suspect there will be a few poorly-trained, unsophisticated clowns out there calling themselves "hypnotherapists" who are actually doing little more than that, and wondering why their practice isn't doing very well. Sometimes medical people like GPs, or perhaps psychotherapists, will have 'experimented' with hypnosis in this way, with a minimum of formal hypnotherapy training - or none - just out of curiosity really, and ended up concluding that success with hypnosis is patchy or disappointing (just like Sigmund Freud did), when in reality they are just conducting it in a very clumsy way because they are misunderstanding it to begin with.

Success with hypnotherapy isn't about getting people to go into trance, that's the easiest thing in the world for anyone who truly understands hypnosis. If any therapist is struggling to get anyone to adopt a trance state, then they do not properly understand hypnosis, it is as simple as that. But if you want the mind to *respond* to suggestion, simply knowing how to 'hypnotize' people is of very little use, in itself. You have to know just what to say to that particular person. In trance or out of trance, the human mind *interprets* things it hears, then either relates to that or ignores it, depending upon how that person feels about that suggestion at that particular moment.

If you want to understand how an expert uses waking suggestion, think about the best courtroom drama you have ever seen, in which a brilliant barrister saves the day by presenting a case so effectively that it wins over not just one individual, but a whole jury – perhaps even the whole courtroom. This is never achieved with a single suggestion, although it may culminate in one. First the groundwork is laid, and it takes time. The barrister is patient, he knows what he is about, and where he is headed, but probably no-one else does. This is his particular talent: to see well ahead, to organise many different aspects of the case, to anticipate the counter-arguments and the objections, to know the other possible viewpoints and deal with all of them, to make sure there are no hitches. Or if something unexpected arises, to be able to think on his feet and turn it to a positive use if possible, or else get around it somehow.

In hypnotherapy it does not have to be that dramatic, because therapy is a one-to-one situation where there is no need to *project*, to perform like that or 'work the room', as the barrister may feel it necessary to do. No, it is much more low-key, but every bit as effective, as complex preparations are built-in to the conversational discussion that precedes the trance. We call that discussion "the pre-talk", and it is as much a part of the hypnotherapy process as the trance experience, although clients are usually unaware of that fact. Waking suggestion plays a key role.

Perhaps a detailed example would be useful here, to understand how this functions in practice. During the pre-talk, whilst I am explaining to the client all about the Subconscious mind I include a number of comments that sound as if they are just informative, but are actually aimed at improving their response in trance. One of the questions we are often asked by clients is: "How will you get through to my Subconscious? How can you get it to respond?" This question reveals a common anxiety: clients are assuming that it will be *difficult* to get the Subconscious to change something through the hypnotherapy process, simply because they cannot make that change happen by themselves. After all, it's their mind, isn't it? So if they cannot do it, how on earth am I going to achieve this? That is what is puzzling them, because of course they are new to hypnotherapy and don't realise that it is actually very easy, provided what I am suggesting is genuinely in line with what they want as an outcome.

So to set their minds at rest, whether they personally ask that question or not, I explain to all clients, usually just before we get into the trance section of the session:

> "...that the Subconscious is very easy to work with, because it is goal-driven and always aims to succeed, so it 'wants to help'. I point out that the conscious mind is different, because it already thinks this is a difficult matter, simply because the conscious mind itself cannot change it. Also, from about the age of three or four we are beginning to realise that not everything we are told is true, so we begin to filter information mentally to see if we think it is true or not, based upon what we have already learned. This gradually develops into a healthy skepticism in the conscious mind, which is necessary to protect us from the lies and trickery we may encounter in the world around us. This means that the conscious mind will always listen to new information with *due skepticism*, whatever other attitudes it may also have (eg. interest, curiosity, hope).
>
> The Subconscious mind on the other hand never develops skepticism because the conscious mind has already done that, so that line of defence is already in place. Also, the Subconscious mind does not really bother with the world around us anyway most of the time, that is really the conscious mind's job. Therefore, during the discussion part of the session when I am explaining everything to the client's conscious

mind, it is likely to consider what I am saying with due skepticism, and may not believe it is going to work. But when I am talking to the Subconscious during the trance section, it has a completely different attitude. It doesn't listen with skepticism at all, but takes a much more practical view: it listens to see if this sounds like a good idea. And if it sounds like a good idea to the Subconscious, then it will simply do it – not because the therapist says so, but because it is obviously a good idea, isn't it? Which makes it very easy to work with the Subconscious mind (I tell the client), because I only need to set out a clear case for why this change would be full of advantages for you, and just be honest and straightforward about the details and your Subconscious will take the opportunity to take care of that for you."

Now, I am not misleading the client in any way because all of that is true enough. But the client may be under the impression I am simply *talking about* the Subconscious. In reality, if you look back over those last two paragraphs they are absolutely loaded with 'waking' suggestions. Most of them are also what we would call *embedded* suggestions, because they are not immediately noticeable *as* suggestions. This becomes clearer if we contrast embedded suggestions with *direct* ones, such as: "From this moment on, you will not feel the slightest desire to eat crisps!" which is obvious enough to the client as a suggestion. On the face of it, the statements embedded with waking suggestions sound as if I am simply explaining that the conscious mind is skeptical but the Subconscious is more practical, more positive - as if I am just reassuring the client that the Subconscious is likely to respond even if they have conscious doubts.

We need to unpack the text to find the actual suggestions.

The first paragraph is really about the conscious mind, but begins with a simple statement about the Subconscious which includes these embedded suggestions: <u>the Subconscious</u>: very easy to work with... goal driven... aims to succeed... wants to help...

Then I acknowledge and validate the skepticism in the conscious mind, explaining *why* the conscious mind "*thinks* this is difficult" - an expression which suggests it is normal to *think* that, but implies it is happily a misunderstanding, which it is. Then I point to the normal development and purpose of "healthy skepticism" in a way that suggests skepticism is not a problem at all, but actually a positive, useful thing that "protects <u>us</u>" from the lies and trickery in the world. This suggestion unites *us* (myself and the client) *against* lies and trickery *out there*, as opposed to in here, where there isn't any. Then, by listing other, more positive attitudes the conscious mind could adopt (interest, curiosity, hope) I place these against skepticism as alternatives, so that these can replace skepticism as the dominant conscious outlook, or at least balance it. Not all suggestion in hypnotherapy is aimed at the Subconscious.

Having embraced the doubts and uncertainties of the conscious mind and reassured the client that these attributes are normal, and useful in other contexts, we can place all that aside and move back to the Subconscious for the second batch of embedded 'waking' suggestions:

<u>the Subconscious</u>: never develops skepticism... more practical... it listens... sounds like a good idea(1)... sounds like a good idea(2)... obviously a good idea(3)... very easy to work with... clear case for change... full of advantages for you... honest and straightforward... take the opportunity... will take care of that.

Now, just look at how much positive 'waking' suggestion was loaded into that short, two-paragraph section about the attitude of the Subconscious. It only takes about 90 seconds to say – two minutes at the outside – but to anyone who might have been worried about how I was going to get their Subconscious to respond, that is a very influential and reassuring two minutes. Don't forget, all this happens before any formal trance procedure is even begun so the client does not view it *as* suggestion, but as information, and very welcome information too. Therefore they are highly likely to accept that as fact, and even though I do not control that choice, if I present those details in a very acceptable form which they should have no particular reason to question, then the effect is reassuring. You see, I am about to present this person with a convincing case for freedom from tobacco. I want them to go into that feeling *reassured,* not doubtful and anxious, and that is the main aim of the 'waking' suggestions detailed above.

Two minutes, that is all the time it took to do that. The vast majority of hypnotherapy sessions I conduct are two hours in length. One hour of chat, one hour relaxing in a comfy chair with eyes closed. In a smoking session the trance section consists of me talking rapidly and virtually non-stop, and the amount of positive suggestion coded into that is phenomenal. It would takes months to go through every detail of all that in the way I just did with the two paragraphs quoted as an example.

In addition to that, in the pre-talk I am usually speaking for about 70% of the time, as I explain everything, and a great deal of what I say is actually constructed in that way, geared to creating that kind of reassurance and change. I don't mean it is scripted, that is just the way I organise language now when I'm working, it has become second nature. It is really the culmination of thousands of hours conducting hypnotherapy sessions, coupled with a deep interest in language and suggestion. And also in *people* – how they think, how they feel. Anyone who doesn't have a really keen interest in human beings is never going to be much of a hypnotherapist.

## "I've had hypnotherapy before, but..."

I would now like to invite you to consider a conversation I have had with clients on numerous occasions:

"I'm a bit worried, I'm not sure if this is going to work because you see I've had hypnotherapy once before, about ten years ago and nothing happened... in fact I never went 'under', so I felt the whole thing was... "

"A waste of time?"

"Well, yes – I mean, no disrespect to you of course but when I went to see that chap it just seemed as if nothing was really happening, and it just had no effect at all, really."

"I see!"

"And I just wondered if that meant, you know, I can't be hypnotised, because not everybody can, can they? I thought maybe I'm just not susceptible... but I really want to get rid of this problem, so I thought I might just give it another go, you know."

"Okay. Can I just ask, how many sessions did you have, back then?"

"Oh, just the one – I was supposed to have another, but I didn't really see the point." [N.B. Some clients may report having had two or three, but in effect they were all just as pointless as the first, for reasons I will explain in a moment.]

"Well that's understandable, but might I just ask: how long were you actually with the therapist, in that first session?"

"Oh... a bit less than an hour... forty, maybe fifty minutes altogether."

"Ah. And how much did the therapist explain to you about hypnotherapy before getting on to the trance part?"

"Well very little, really – we just talked about the problem for a bit, and then he asked me if I had any questions. Then he started with all the relaxation stuff, but I never really felt very relaxed, to be honest."

"Right. And what was the place like? How did you feel about this person, anyway?"

"Well I thought he was a bit odd, really! I mean he never actually looked at me when I was talking, and seemed hardly to be listening to what I was saying sometimes. And the room was cold - and smelled of cats, and I'm a bit scared of cats..."

OK, let's just sum that up, shall we?

1. Nowhere near enough session-time set aside for the client's needs.
2. No explanation of hypnosis or the Subconscious, so the client is left with all the typical misunderstandings of hypnosis: "under", "susceptible", "cannot be hypnotised" etc.
3. No waking suggestion utilised whatsoever.
4. Uncomfortable environment.
5. Odd, distant therapist.
6. Cold, smelly room.
7. Fear of cats.

Just how much positive response would that have got out of anybody?

Clearly, this is not a failure of hypnotherapy as a therapeutic mode, but a complete failure on the part of the 'therapist' to carry out any sort of useful hypnotherapy in the first place. Now replace the "odd hypnotherapist" in that scenario with an "odd psychologist", leave all the other factors the same, and you would get the same outcome: zero positive response. Now try an odd psychiatrist, an odd psychoanalyst, an odd counsellor. Makes no difference to the outcome, because the therapist's negligence and unprofessionalism created a negative mindset in the client. The therapist could have attempted to use anything from NLP to voodoo, from crystals to ear-candles, none of it would have got a positive response out of that client on the day because of everything else that was bothering her!

Given that any *one* of those negative factors can stall a hypnotherapy session, it follows that care and diligence, sensitivity and attention to detail are all important for the successful hypnotherapist – just as they would be for the surgeon, the pilot, the dentist and many other experts in whose care we may find ourselves at one time or another. Those professionals too, if they are really expert and taking proper care of the people in their charge, will be using 'waking' suggestion to great effect, whether they know it or not:

"It's really a very routine surgical procedure I've successfully conducted many times before..."

"We have some interesting weather coming up, but we should be sailing through that in a little under ten minutes... our descent will be smooth and easy, and it's a beautiful day in Majorca!"

And here's one my dentist came out with recently when I was having a tooth capped for the first time. The whole thing had taken quite a while and was a bit uncomfortable, but he made it all okay just as he got to the end of the procedure, by muttering: "You see, if you take the time... to do these things properly... in the first place... then they should be... (just bite down again for me? That's it)... then they should be good... and sound ...and solid... (there we go!) ...for fifteen years or more."

A true professional, just what I needed to hear.

## The Other Side of the Coin

In reality we are all being presented with waking suggestion many times throughout the day. All advertising is waking suggestion for a start. Some things that people say to each other can function as waking suggestion, and in certain professions a proper appreciation of this should be built into the training right from the start. Teachers and medical people especially need an expert understanding of the likely effects of suggestion, not just to help those in their care more effectively but to avoid doing lasting damage through sheer carelessness and ignorance.

Of course, some negative waking suggestion is deliberate, calculated and malicious. Many readers will be able to recall, for example, a moment when a teacher put them down in front of a whole class – or even a whole school – in a way that was obviously ruthless and intended to be devastating to their self-esteem. Any memory like that which still makes you wince when you think about it had its full effect at the time, and is still 'radioactive' as it were, still emitting negativity deep in the Subconscious mind.

Recently I was told by a stroke victim that she had been recovering some movement and feeling in her left side progressively, right up until the day when she asked her consultant how long it would take to get back the full use of her arm. His reply was delivered with such certainty and such a complete lack of sensitivity that it put her in shock:

"You'll never get it back."

My client told me that she just stared at him with her mouth open. The word she used to describe her reaction to that was "devastated". Her recovery stopped right there. Shock is a *trance state*. Right then and there her tentative recovery was utterly defeated: she was unfortunately convinced by the *mere suggestion* that she would never get back the use of her arm, and all the hope and motivation she had had for the recovery process before that was destroyed in a moment.

Now, you might be thinking: "Well, I wouldn't have accepted that! I would have immediately thought: 'I'll show you, pal! That's all you know!'"

The thing is: that is your conscious mind talking. Also, you probably aren't trying to come to terms right now with having had a stroke, which tends to make people feel very vulnerable and uncertain about all sorts of things. Finally, although your conscious mind might, or might not take up that position, being in shock at the time means that the Subconscious is taking all this in as well, and if the Subconscious fear that it might be true outweighs the hope that it isn't – as it would in many people, I'm afraid – then you're screwed anyway.

Would the lady concerned have recovered any further if the consultant had never said that? We don't know. Some might even argue that the consultant had a duty to tell her that, if that was his honest opinion. I could not disagree more, since a consultant would have to be infallible to justify that, and no-one is. What we do know for sure is that before the consultation she regarded herself as in recovery, making progress and expecting to get back the use of her arm. As we say in hypnotherapy: "What the mind expects tends to be realised". There was, at the very least, a chance for that to happen. So he took that hope and positive expectation and just dashed it to the ground. What an idiot. Simply because he was the 'consultant', the medical expert, she had no grounds for rejecting the suggestion, so she left the room honestly believing all hope was lost. Four years later, in my office, she told me that her recovery had not progressed at all since that day.

"No problem," you might think, "because surely the expert hypnotherapist can simply hypnotise the client and remove the negative suggestion, replacing it with a much more positive suggestion about the recovery getting underway again!"

After four years? Haven't those four years of stagnation just confirmed what the consultant predicted? Don't forget, for a positive suggestion to be wholeheartedly accepted it has to strike the client's Subconscious mind as 'acceptable', i.e. something which can be believed. You can bet I presented exactly that case to her in the trance part of her session, and I did it with the utmost conviction. To do anything less would be to let her down. But when it comes to responding positively, we have to recognise that she was seriously 'challenged' as they say. After all, wasn't she really only consulting me now out of desperation? That's not a positive mental state, and positive mental states are kind of important when it comes to getting positive change accepted and acted upon in hypnotherapy. And in any case, who was the expert on strokes in her estimation: myself or her damn consultant? Who am I to be challenging his original prognosis? Finally, if you put yourself in her position all these years later, wouldn't the prospect of recovery *beginning again* seem nothing short of miraculous?

I have no information on how that lady is today. As I write this, the session I'm referring to took place only about three weeks ago, so it is a bit soon to be following that up anyway – but these are the cases where I only do what the client has asked me to do - I don't make any promises or predictions of any kind. That's the mistake the consultant made. He promised her she would never recover the use of her left arm. Of course the hypnotherapist has no right to promise that she will recover the use of her arm, and I didn't. But I would also argue that the consultant had no right to assure her that she wouldn't, and those of us who understand the significance of belief in the Subconscious field know that there is a serious possibility that he actually scuppered her recovery quite unnecessarily.

<u>Just a Suggestion:</u> If that was the best contribution her consultant had to offer, I'd say she would have been better off without him. Why did he bother coming in off the golf course just to tell her that? Is that medical help? As an example of negative waking suggestion that is so much worse than useless that I think the guy should do all his patients a favour and just stay on the golf course. In all weathers. And when it gets a bit stormy, I suggest that he should raise up his putter, hold it high above his head and wait...

...until he finds out for himself what a devastating shock feels like.

## Some Useful Laws of Hypnotherapy

1. The outcome of any hypnotherapy session is not determined by the hypnotist, but by the reaction, on that day, of the Subconscious mind of the client. The hypnotist has no control over that factor at all, and in fact can only hope to influence the Subconscious mind's choices by the strength of the case for change he is presenting for consideration.
2. The Subconscious mind of the client is not affected in any way by the conscious opinions of the client. The Subconscious has complete freedom to make its own decisions, and has its own agenda.
3. It is normal and usual for the conscious mind of the client to be astonished by positive changes after hypnotherapy, because the conscious mind was not really expecting that,

especially if the person never experienced hypnotherapy before.

This is largely because the conscious mind does not really believe in the Subconscious, except perhaps in theory. N.B. Since this factor is an effect of culture and education, it is not set in stone. This lack of conscious understanding could be completely resolved by building a proper understanding of the Subconscious mind into education and culture. This would effectively make everybody - compared to the way we are today – seem Superhuman. In truth it is only our actual potential, made real by removing the various ordinary bars that stymie us. (Now *there's* a word you don't get to trot out very often!)

At present, though, not only does the conscious mind not really believe in the Subconscious, by extension it does not usually believe in hypnotherapy either. Except perhaps in theory.

4. For an excellent response to be elicited, *it does not matter* what the conscious mind believes, or does not believe, either at the outset or during the therapy process.
5. What does matter is the mood of the client, their emotional take on the proceedings or the issue at hand. If this is forward-looking and positive, the client's response is likely to be positive. If it is backward-looking and negative, or oppositional, then the response will be poorer, or there may be no positive response at all.

The skill of an expert hypnotherapist is to help the client to establish the most positive mood possible before trance-work begins, and during trance-work, to incline the client's Subconscious towards moving on and change - as preferable to stasis, stagnation and frustration.

6. How much a person responds during any hypnotherapy session is directly proportional to what they want, expect and accept – on an *emotional,* not an *analytical* level - within the session.

One of the things that can get in the way of this is simple *fear of failure*. Sometimes it is necessary to clear this fear of failure before you can get anywhere with anything else.

7. The Subconscious controls, to the finest detail, all emotions and understands them completely. It can change any of them in any degree, at any time, simply upon request - much to the amazement of the conscious mind. Actually the conscious mind should not really be amazed by this, since the Subconscious reviews feelings anyway as we go through life, and adjusts them from time to time according to its own preferences.

When people say: "I can't help the way I *feel*, can I?" (as if their feelings were controlled by somebody else) that is the conscious mind talking - freely admitting that it does not control emotions. This is because the Subconscious is the emotional centre, it controls and operates all emotional drives, including the ones we are not even consciously aware of but which are influencing our choices and behaviour anyway. The conscious mind is under the impression that emotions simply *are what they are* and cannot change, because it doesn't know about the role of the Subconscious. This limitation can of course be overcome, via the learning process that is hypnotherapy.

## Erroneous Beliefs

At the centre of the word *believe,* is the word 'lie'. Lies or misunderstandings are often at the centre of beliefs, but not always of course. The trouble is, as long as you believe something is true in reality, you cannot see the **lie** (or error) at the centre of it. Fortunately this distinction is more of a concern to the conscious mind than the Subconscious, because:

8. The Subconscious mind is not unduly concerned with objective truth, but is goal-driven. The idea that there is

such a thing as Universal Truth is a conscious notion. In the Subconscious mind there is no obvious difference between reality and fantasy; neither is privileged, they count for the same. Only the conscious mind creates a distinction. I use the term "creates" because truth is actually a construction, though the conscious mind usually prefers to deny that.

## Pick a Truth, any Truth...

To recognise this as fact we only have to observe how many different things are held to be true by different people at any one time. They cannot all be right, can they? Yet none of us think that we ourselves are wrong, we think that all those who think otherwise are wrong. But we cannot all be right about that either, which inevitably proves that many of us currently believe things that are not true but we honestly think that we are the ones who are right. Yet unbeknown to us we are unjustly judging someone else to be wrong when in fact they are quite correct, we simply haven't realised that to be the case.

Don't be surprised if you find that last bit hard to believe in your own case. Unless of course you doubt yourself a lot, for then you will find it really easy to believe and probably suspected it anyway. This doesn't mean you were right, by the way, it only proves that your doubts were valid enough, just not necessarily conclusive. Still it is reassuring to know that you weren't just doubting yourself for no reason, is it not? I mean who wants to finds themselves suspecting a thing like that? Surely any sane person would rather feel absolutely certain that there was sound reason for their self-doubt, otherwise they might find it difficult to keep undermining and questioning themselves all the time... which might lead to self-assuredness, or confidence or something.

It is also worth pointing out that some of the things we used to believe we would now regard as ignorant or naive, and so we find that we have at some point apparently accepted as 'true enough' things to which we used to feel inclined to object. Hence it becomes clear that beliefs can function as normal without truth even being involved, though we usually think it is central to them. This despite the fact that the only thing visibly and undeniably at the centre of beliefs is 'lie'. (Quite fun this, isn't it? No? Then allow me to recommend *Change Your Life In 7 Days* by Paul McKenna. He's a hypnotist too, you know. As is Sooty. I believe that I mentioned in Volume One that I have nothing against either of them. Especially Sooty.)

## Where were we?

9. It is an ongoing project of the conscious mind to establish a thing called "truth", and then support the construction by continually distinguishing it from any notions or meanings that fall outside of that construction. The conscious mind sometimes regards these matters as being very important. For the Subconscious however, truth is everywhere and nowhere and it really isn't a problem.

This fact is clear from our experiences of dreaming. Whilst we are asleep the conscious analytical mind is resting. Dreaming is pure Subconscious thought, and so in a dream any mad thing can be experienced as real, without even appearing unlikely or bizarre. Later, when the conscious mind analyses any part of the dream after waking, a distinction between "real" and "imaginary" details can be drawn. But whilst asleep – i.e. in free Subconscious thought – anything can be accepted as real experience, no matter how wild or ludicrous it is compared to external (waking) reality.

## When the conscious mind is struggling

Failures of the conscious mind to properly or consistently distinguish real from unreal are labelled variously as forms of 'psychoses' (or disorders) in the mind sciences. For hypnotherapy, which is *not* a 'mind science' but the practical art of meta-communication, these are often - especially in milder cases - issues of perception rather than pathology. In other words, hypnotherapy can often eliminate them entirely if therapy goes well.

Serious mental illness, conversely, is outside the scope of hypnotherapy usually. This is not because hypnotherapy would be no use in the treatment of serious mental illness – it was certainly of great importance in the work of the American psychiatrist Milton Erickson – but rather because private hypnotherapy practitioners are not psychiatrists. We are not trained or experienced in the details of mental illnesses, nor are we medical practitioners so we do not work with people who are seriously mentally ill. We *do* normally work with anxiety, mental stress, unhappiness and various forms of mental distress, but these are not abnormal states. They are perfectly normal reactions under given circumstances, such as anyone may be prone to if conditions were sufficiently negative. Whereas, say, believing you are Napoleon or dearly wanting to stab anyone dressed as Santa Claus would not be.

## **Movements in the Unseen** (or, orchestral manoeuvres in the dark)

10. Conducting a hypnotherapy session is like conducting a magnificent orchestra, but with numerous scores, some of which the conductor has never seen.

I'll just run that one by you again. Conducting a hypnotherapy session is like conducting a magnificent orchestra (the mind of another human being – and do remember that the conductor is only a guiding figure, every element of the orchestra is freely controlling itself) ...but with numerous scores (the life-experiences, issues, beliefs and *intentions* of that person - both conscious and Subconscious) ...some of which, the conductor knows nothing about. This last factor is inevitable because there are always going to be many aspects of a client's experiences that never come up in the sessions, yet may have significance regarding the issues we are addressing.

Given all that, some might think: "Well that's impossible! How could you ever get *anywhere?*" But you see, as long as you're working *with* that person's mind and not *on* it, you can get just as far as that person feels like going. Their Subconscious mind knows the whole story, you see.

Why do they need a third party, then? Why can't that person do it all by themselves? Well, firstly because their conscious mind is likely to know very little about their own Subconscious, so it tends to be limited to self-referential lines of thought in its own processing, and secondly because the change process is difficult to both *instigate* and *respond to* all by yourself. Therapy is a dynamic process and the best way to proceed is via a live, unscripted, genuinely spontaneous one-to-one event. Try to do that all by yourself and it is probably going to be a non-event.

11. Subconscious World - or life as perceived by the Subconscious mind - is quite another mental dimension, made up of myriad kaleidoscopic reflections of the external world - which is pretty interesting in itself, but which becomes something else again in the world of the Imagination, where everything is possible and ideas become potentially infinite. Add the fact that no two minds have ever consisted of exactly the same combination of consistent factors, and the imaginative potential of the whole species becomes absolutely phenomenal. Hence the astonishing technical brilliance of the human race. Our analytical power is good, but it is

pedestrian compared to our imaginative power, which is always way, way ahead of our actual technical accomplishments but hauls them on, breathlessly, at breakneck speed. The human race is run at such a pace that we are almost unable to keep up with the accelerating velocity of our dreams and ambitions. The conscious mind's analytical powers are utterly outclassed in Subconscious World, which means that this mental territory cannot be mapped. Any attempt to define or organise Subconscious World would be like herding cats, so those seekers of knowledge who have a scientific approach to learning would need to adjust to that caveat before they could really start to get anywhere. Even those of us who function as a 'guide' in Subconscious World are not referring to a map. Instead it would be more appropriate to say that we just travel in it. Every journey is unique.

It is not surprising that people of an analytical and scientific mindset feel rather lost in the field of hypnotherapy, or attempt to impose some sort of 'order' upon it, which is always reductive and seriously lacking in insight because it is formulated within the 'little fort' from which conscious perception peeps out.

Subconscious World is Dreamland: the beyond of known, possible and proven. What really worries the analytical type, when it comes to considering the Subconscious mind, what makes them feel uneasy is that conscious analytical powers are not very useful in Dreamland. The analyst's way is subverted here, as Lewis Carroll rather brilliantly dramatised whenever he had Alice attempt to use reason in her various arguments with the characters in Wonderland. It simply doesn't get her anywhere, and she is clearly frustrated by that. Just like Alice, the analytical type of thinker will tend to object to the different forms of thought and the 'play' in meaning, and perhaps feel indignant about the fact that logic and rationality have no special status in the field of the Subconscious mind. They are *understood* by the

Subconscious, incidentally – it is just not bound by them. This irritates the type of dogged analytical thinker who would prefer it if *everything* were bound by logic and reason - despite the fact that this would make the world so joyless and boring that we would all end up buying shotguns so that we could blow our boring, joyless brains out. Or maybe just theirs.

This Subconscious subversion of logic and rationality is sometimes regarded as actually being *dangerous* by some of the more vehement analytical types, but to be fair to analytical people generally most of them don't find the random generator of ideas that is the Subconscious mind threatening in any way. It is, in truth, every bit as capable of producing ideas that are universally appreciated as genius as it is capable of producing nonsense and silliness. And that is something that could truly be said of the conscious mind as well!

You can see a perfect example of the futility of conscious attempts to map Subconscious World in the Freudian attempts to interpret dreams, and all the nonsense that produced before the project was generally given up as a bad job. Once you decide, for example, that dreaming of a house equates to a symbolic representation of the body (or indeed anything else in particular) you are being reductive, closing down other subjective meanings and boxing it off - as if Subconscious thought "needs sorting out". To anyone truly familiar with the field of the Subconscious mind this is a rather amusing notion: that the poor little conscious mind could genuinely appreciate the depth and complexity, the power and magnificence of the Subconscious. But in any case, interpretation simply isn't necessary. Dreams have their own role. Stripping them down and rebuilding them under conscious direction is just a waste of time – as indeed we all recognise immediately when somebody else is telling us about their dreams. So boring and meaningless on a *conscious* level, in fact, that it is a struggle even to listen politely.

This does not indicate that dreams are meaningless by the way, but that the conscious mind should mind its own business. Stick to what it is good at, dealing with the outside world and other people in the here and now. The conscious mind does not understand dreaming because it is Subconscious thought, and the conscious mind just does not think that way. Interpreting dreams with conscious logic is like translating Shakespeare into hieroglyphs. So much would be lost in translation it is a completely pointless exercise.

Having said all that, the *mood* pervading the dream may be a useful indicator of Subconscious concerns of the moment - just as Alice's changing moods and feelings are what really stir her into action, and then the nonsense of the conversations becomes incidental. In dreams, the detail can be pointing the right way or the wrong way, but the mood will tend to be the more reliable indicator of the overall Subconscious direction of travel.

12. The word "hypnosis", as it is commonly used is almost completely misleading because the subject is so very much misunderstood by the vast majority of people. What most people think of as hypnosis does not really exist. Hypnotherapy, as a process, must *always* begin with clearing the client's misconceptions about hypnosis. One day this may no longer be necessary but unfortunately I will not live to see that, which means I will probably have to spend the rest of my professional life explaining what hypnosis is not, several times a day. Neglecting to do this is quite likely to undermine the effectiveness of the session, although in some cases it might not. One of the curious things about hypnotherapy is that even if it is conducted rather poorly, it can still sometimes be perfectly successful. This is really because the client manifests the outcome, not the hypnotist, but of course a good response is more likely with a well-conducted session.

# The All-Important 13th Law:

There *are no laws* in hypnosis really - and consequently no lawmen. (Hurrah!) Thought exceeds reality and the physical world, and it can never be restricted by legislation or policed. Dreams and daydreams are free-thought-revelry, the origin of all new things, the outriders at every kind of frontier, the most surprising and elusive of all experience. This is the particular field of human existence in which hypnotherapy moves.

# How to Choose a Good Hypnotherapist

Therapists often specialise in different issues, have different training and use various methods, so it is a question of finding one that suits you. If you want to stop smoking you should seek a therapist who specialises in that issue - and most of these will now be approaching smoking cessation as a one-session procedure. This does not mean everybody will respond immediately, but that most will. The ones who need a further session, or a later session because they started again, have not failed – see *Relapse is not Failure* in Section 14 - they simply need a further session. It is quite normal that some people will need more than one session.

However, if any hypnotherapist tells you in advance that it will take several sessions to stop you smoking, my advice would be to look elsewhere. Although none of us can *promise* smoking cessation in one session, that outcome certainly can be achieved in the majority of cases presenting for private therapy. No hypnotherapist should be guessing, in advance, how many sessions anything might take because it can be nothing more than a guess. If all clients are told – for example – that it will take three sessions, very few of them would then stop during the first session, obviously. It is all too easy for a therapist to create expectations of slower change by suggesting that – and therefore slower change in reality - than the client might otherwise have achieved. Any change process should be taken a session at a time, and it is up to the client to decide how many sessions they need, not the therapist.

## Sound Recordings offered as 'therapy'

Sometimes people think they've already tried hypnotherapy because they bought a 'hypnosis' tape or CD, then they lay on their bed and listened to it, perhaps a few times. That is nowhere near as effective as real hypnotherapy. I don't mean such things are completely useless, just that they would probably prove fairly useless to most people especially if they have never had the dynamics of hypnotherapy explained to them in detail. This is because they would not know how to create the right mood and frame of mind for themselves in which to *respond,* and of course they cannot ask any specific questions.

Some therapists sell tapes and CDs, and some make a tape recording of the session and give that to the client. These can be of some limited use, especially if the client has been told how to respond to it, and then they actually go ahead and *do* that. But if someone just buys a "Cure your Fear of Flying" CD off the shelf, knowing little about hypnotherapy or how to respond to the recorded suggestions, then they probably will not notice much change, if any.

Having said that, there will always be a few people who happen to respond quite well despite the various shortcomings of this approach. For the majority though, it is much better to forget recordings and have a proper session. After all, the human mind is a living thing, it responds much better to another living being than a recording. Especially a recording made by a person you have never met, who is not speaking to you personally anyway but into a recording machine, which tends to make their speech a little unnatural and uninspiring – even false. The Subconscious is nothing short of brilliant when it comes to matters of communication: it picks up on subtle things like that and is not impressed. In other words, you are likely to remain unmoved by the experience.

## Effective, one-to-one therapy

A good session with an expert will probably not be brief. Hypnotherapy often clears issues very quickly, in terms of the number of sessions needed, but the process itself is not quick. It is quite unlike stage hypnosis in this respect. Stage hypnosis can be very rapid in practice, because confusing the conscious mind is an important element in it (just like in a magic trick), and because they are going for immediate reactions rather than permanent change.

That is not usually how we conduct effective hypnotherapy. Clients have sometimes told me they have been to see a hypnotherapist on some previous occasion but were only there for about half an hour. My advice would be that if a hypnotherapist has not got much time for you, then that is not the therapist for you. There is no ideal session length, but anything much under an hour is questionable, especially for a first session. Personally I set two hours aside for every session, no matter what it is for. You can get a lot done in two hours.

I am frequently asked, especially by email from people in other cities or countries, how a person should go about finding a good therapist. Just because somebody has done a basic course and learned about hypnotic states, that doesn't make them a talented therapist. In the public imagination, if a person knows how to "hypnotise" a smoker, then they assume that the hypnotist ought to be able to stop the smoker smoking – as if hypnotising them was the important bit. Once upon a time this used to be a common demonstration in stage shows, in the days when smoking was still allowed in the auditorium. The stage hypnotist could easily get the smoker to suddenly react quite differently to smoke by suggesting it will taste like burning rubber or something like that. As a stunt this can be quite dramatic, but what the public don't realise is that such a simple aversion suggestion would only have a temporary effect for the majority of smokers. Stopping smoking permanently with hypnotherapy is much more detailed and complex than that, but that does not mean it is difficult. For a talented and experienced therapist it is easy enough. For the smoker it is effortless.

## Selecting Your Therapist

If you can get a personal recommendation from someone who has already been successful with a particular therapist, this is usually a good choice although it has to be said that rapport is still important, you have to be able to get along with that therapist yourself. If you have no recommendation, seek out a few local options from classified or online directories and ring around.

When you make initial enquiries, do not book. Always say you have a few more people to ring, and that you will call back. If a therapist tries to talk you into booking even when you seemed reluctant to do so, do not book with them. If they talk you into it somehow and you feel as if you were pressured into that decision, phone them back and cancel. Go with someone else. Or if you don't feel like cancelling, just don't turn up - it will serve them right for pressuring you. There's no come-back, they cannot force you to pay for the session or anything like that. If they try to tell you otherwise, there's your confirmation that they care more about your money than they care about you. No talented, successful hypnotherapist will ever push you into booking a session - they would never need to do that because their services are always in demand. The last thing you need is a pushy, self-centred therapist.

Make sure you get to speak to the therapist, not some assistant. Avoid booking a session until you have spoken to the person you will be seeing. Prepare some questions beforehand, and have them written down so you don't just go blank when the conversation starts. Use the questions to get the therapist talking.

Do they seem easy to get along with? Helpful, friendly, considerate? Do they sound confident, trustworthy, encouraging, supportive? Ask them what they do, how it works, what they think will be necessary to solve your problem. The purpose of this is not so much to get the answers to those questions but to get some measure of what kind of a person you are dealing with here and whether you get the feeling they can help *you*. Their qualifications alone will not tell you important things like this. See if you like them when you talk to them, that is probably more important than how many certificates they have on their wall. Trust your gut feeling on this one, and if communication doesn't seem so easy for you when talking to that therapist, try ringing another! Hypnotherapy is all about communication, and the rapport should be pretty easy right from the start.

## Masculine and Feminine Types

It is helpful to know that therapists can be roughly divided into two types which we in the profession term masculine and feminine. It is not a simple matter of gender, but of style and approach. I think it is fair to say that most hypnotherapists are likely to be on the 'feminine' side, which means that their style will be gentle, supportive, understanding, patient and kindly. Those who might be regarded as 'masculine' would be more forthright, less indulgent, more commanding and abrupt in their approach. These are generalisations, but it is helpful to be aware of them. If you had a domineering parent you would find it difficult to respond positively to a 'masculine' therapist, but a 'feminine' one would be fine. If on the other hand your parents were wishy-washy, and it drove you crazy – and especially if you have spent years in the army or one of the emergency services and respond better to being given clear instructions by someone who is confident about taking charge - you might do well with a more 'masculine' therapist. See how you feel about their attitude when you talk to them on the phone.

## Tele-phobia

For some people telephoning is a bit traumatic in itself. I understand this, because I used to feel that way when I was young. I lacked confidence when telephoning anyone I didn't already know and tended to avoid it. If you feel like that, you could ask someone who is happy to chat away on the phone to ring around for you, preferably a good 'people person' who can get the measure of someone by just talking to them. Also, you can find out more about a therapist from perusing their website, if they have one. You might prefer to use email for enquiries rather than use the phone, especially if you usually communicate that way. Do bear in mind though that emails and text messages are notoriously poor ways of communicating anything except simple details like dates and times. Misunderstandings can easily occur, and the less of that there is the better, obviously.

## The Rest is Effortless!

In the entire process of utilising hypnotherapy services, actually telephoning or emailing to make an appointment is probably the only part that might seem daunting or difficult in any way. Once that is done, if you then feel glad you have booked the session, then that is a good sign. If on the other hand you find that you feel worried about it afterwards, just consider this: are you simply worried about your issue, or whether you have chosen the right therapist?

If you are just worried about the issue and whether or not the therapy is going to work, that's perfectly normal and you should proceed as planned. But if you have doubts about your choice of therapist, ask yourself this: are you worried just because you are usually uncertain about making decisions and therefore would probably have these worries whoever you had picked? Or is something bothering you about the process of enquiring and booking that particular therapist which you just cannot put your finger on?

If you are just a worrier who routinely doubts their decisions, give yourself a slap and proceed as planned. However, if something deep down is bothering you about that particular therapist, cancel. Or get someone else to do it for you. Your Subconscious mind isn't happy with the choice and you should just find someone else. You don't need to work out why, just trust your gut feeling - that is not the right therapist for you. It doesn't mean there is anything wrong with the therapist necessarily, it is just that we all respond better on a Subconscious level to people we like. You'll get better results with someone you feel fine about.

If you cancel, but the therapist phones you back later to try to talk you round, or betrays any unhappiness about the cancellation, there is your confirmation you were right to trust your Subconscious! Those reactions from a therapist are very unprofessional and may be an indication they are not very busy. Professional experts in hypnotherapy will always accept a cancellation with good grace and thank you for letting them know. This is best practice because the therapist has no idea why the client is really cancelling that appointment, we only know what we are being told. We may have lost an appointment but we haven't necessarily lost the client. They may book in again at a later date, but only if we handle the cancellation with good grace. Also, potential clients may feel uncomfortable about having to cancel at all, and it is our duty to protect them by being kind and understanding. At least they have taken the trouble to let us know, unlike the clients who book a session and just never show up! (See Case Mysteries No. 10: *Mysterious Disappearances.*)

## Directories

There are currently two types of directories: on-line directories and the traditional phone books like Yellow Pages. So many on-line directories have now sprung up that the traditional 'hard copy' phone books are almost certainly on their way out, but as they are still around for the moment I can offer a few useful bits of advice about them.

## The Big Heavy Books

If you don't have a therapist recommended to you, you may find yourself trawling through the classified section of the local telephone directory for a likely-looking practitioner. This can be a bit confusing at first glance, especially in the big cities because there may be too much choice. For example, in my local classified directory which covers the South Manchester area of the U.K. there are about sixty practitioners in the hypnotherapy section. Some just list a phone number, but many have some sort of a display advertisement and you only have to look at a dozen or so to realise that hypnotherapists have a bit of a problem when it comes to advertising. Since we are all broadly doing the same kind of work, it is difficult to create an advert that stands out, making selection difficult for the client.

What is the new client looking for, as they leaf through the local directory? The nearest therapist? Maybe. The cheapest? Not necessarily. The most professional? Now you're talking. The most successful? Yes, and perhaps the most reassuring choice available. So the main thing we therapists have to do is design our advertisement in such a way that it conveys professionalism, success and reassurance to the wavering prospective client. It's as simple as that. So... how do we do that, exactly?

Some therapists list specialities but the trouble with that is, most of them specialise in the same things so it doesn't help the person looking through the ads, even if that is what they are looking for. Some try to stand out by spending more on a large advert, but then some clients might assume that those therapists will probably be more expensive than the rest and not even ring them. But the most confusing thing of all is the wide range of qualifications and professional associations in the hypnotherapy sector. Aiming to reassure the new client that they are properly qualified, therapists' names usually appear with long lists of letters after them, and often under an association banner which you might see repeated a few times in that section, but you will probably see three or four other associations listed as well. The British Society of Clinical Hypnosis, The Hypnotherapy Association, The National Council for Hypnotherapy, The National Hypnopsychotherapy Council, the General Hypnotherapy Standards Council, The National Register of Hypnotherapists and Psychotherapists, and The Hypnotherapy Society to name but a few.

What is the new client to make of this, how do they choose? Why are there so many societies and national councils anyway? Well, the first thing to say is that there is no need, really, to take all this too seriously. The only reason hypnotherapists are trying so hard to reassure prospective clients that they are reputable and professional is because they know you are probably a bit afraid of hypnotism. Maybe you once saw Paul McKenna persuade someone to dance the funky chicken in a stage show, and so all that these qualifications and professional associations are really telling you - as they appear in these advertisements I mean - is that this is a bona fide therapist who will not make you dance the funky chicken. So ring us, and the only dance you'll be doing is the dance of joy because you got rid of your fear of fish, or you calmly passed your final examinations and have finally been allowed to join the Federation of Master Window Cleaners, or whatever. (That really exists, by the way.)

I think all the hypnotherapy societies should get together and form one big Hypnotherapy Society Society (HSS). That would be simpler, but in the meantime don't let any of this bother you when you are looking for a therapist. Here are my tips:

1. No matter how big the ad, don't assume anything about fees. Ask.

2. A few therapists charge far more than the norm. Avoid them.
3. Talk to the therapists themselves, and choose someone you like.
4. Do ring around six or seven possible options. Do not book yet.
5. Book later, when you are comfortable with your decision.

Remember, the only reasons people hesitate to use hypnotherapy are because they are uncertain about 'the unknown', and afraid of not succeeding. This is ridiculous really, because the contents of your mind consist entirely of *what you know*, so how can anything about your mind be unknown to you? It is literally not possible. When I am talking to clients, I am either telling their conscious mind something their Subconscious already knew, or telling the Subconscious something the conscious mind already knew, so the process is simply enlightening and creates mental harmony.

There is nothing to be afraid of in hypnotherapy, not even delayed success because the worst thing that could possibly happen - your worst case scenario - is that you leave the session exactly the way you were when you went in. This is not what usually happens because usually people get the change they wanted, especially if they chose the right therapist for them. But even if they didn't, the worst that could possibly happen is nothing. What have you lost? Nothing! Except a bit of money. But that isn't anything to be afraid of - you waste money all the time, don't you? Just think how much money you wasted over the last year, one way or another. How much helpful therapy and general pampering could you have got for that? You'll never know just how much success you could be enjoying until you get around to trying it for yourself. No need to keep on doing everything the hard way when the Subconscious is always happy to help.

## How to Accept Suggestions Successfully

At first, people don't realise that they have to *accept* suggestions for change to take place. When first encountering hypnotherapy it is quite common for people to spend the trance part of the first session *waiting* to see if it will work, and *wondering* what the outcome will be. This is understandable, but it is not the best frame of mind for successful outcomes.

Although I do explain these points before the trance part of the initial session, not everybody adjusts their mindset accordingly straight away. This factor will vary, especially in first sessions, according to personality types and also the person's mood on that particular day.

One thing that people may find a little confusing at first is that it doesn't much matter what they think (consciously) during the trance experience, it is how they feel deep down inside (emotionally) about the issues and proposed changes that actually has a real bearing on the outcome. Yet creating just the right mood is actually very easy! Simply:

Look forward eagerly to success.

Welcome each suggestion with enthusiasm.

Recognise that these changes are exactly what you want.

Remember, these are not *my* suggestions, they're yours. I'm only *presenting* them to your Subconscious mind for you because there's no way you can do that for yourself.

So don't hesitate, don't question, don't analyse, don't sit on the fence, don't 'wait to see'... forget past failures... forget other people and their ignorant opinions, forget fears, doubts, worries... forget stage hypnosis... Let all that nonsense fade away because that isn't going to get you what you came for!

Simply:

Look forward eagerly to success, and welcome each suggestion with enthusiasm because these changes are exactly what you want.

Now of course, I can tell people to do that but I can't make them do it. That's up to them.

# Section Sixteen

## Stage Hypnosis (part 2)

First of all, I am not a Stage Hypnotist. Never have been, never wanted to be and never likely to want to become one at any time in the future. This is not to say that there is anything wrong with being a Stage Hypnotist you understand, although some people think there is. No, it is because I am a hypnotherapist and that means I get to use my Special Powers for Good, and not...

Some hypnotherapists foam at the mouth when they talk about Stage Hypnosis. Some even argue that it should be banned, and indeed there have been a handful of well-publicised claims over the decades that suggest Stage Hypnosis may involve the odd risk in extraordinary circumstances. I am not going to rubbish those claims, nor re-hash them either but I will explain, as we proceed, the kind of circumstances in which the Stage Hypnotist can be skating on thin ice. These risks can easily be avoided anyway once the hypnotist knows what they are.

Since I believe the very rare risks can easily be avoided I do not believe banning Stage Hypnosis is necessary at all but I do think that Stage Hypnotists should be properly trained (which they usually aren't at the moment), not just in how to do stage shows and demonstrations but all aspects of hypnosis and how the mind actually works. They should also be taught above all else not to humiliate their chosen few once they are up on the stage. Of course Stage Hypnosis involves ridiculous behaviour but it does not have to be offensive, crude or abusive, and indeed was not usually like that anyway until quite recently. The popularity of Stage Hypnosis in the UK has nose-dived in a single decade, partly because some Stage Hypnotists have encouraged cruder and more offensive antics on stage and TV screen than we have seen before.

This slump in popularity should not be a surprise to anyone, since all those involved in entertainment ought to be keenly aware that if you want your audience to *like you*, it is probably not a good idea to destroy their dignity and then stamp all over it. The people who volunteer to take part are members of the audience after all, and even if the antics are amusing to those who did not volunteer, if it begins to look like exploitation or victimization it is going to make the rest of the audience feel uncomfortable later about applauding it, and that is not how you want your audience to feel as they head home after the event. Next time your show rolls into town, they may prefer to stay home. Nobody is offended by silly behaviour, and a good stage show can be genuinely hilarious if it is imaginative and full of harmless fun. This can all be successfully achieved without turning the player into some sort of victim.

Not so very long ago, a good stage performer could fill a large venue in any major town in the UK. Now they could not, and are pretty much reduced to playing much smaller clubs or pubs, or foreign holiday resorts. The other factor that has brought this change about is the handful of legal claims for damages against stage hypnotists. Even though they very rarely win any kind of ruling against the hypnotist since most of these claims are really unfounded and based on ignorance, they have nevertheless made insurers jumpy, and it is now rather expensive to get cover for hypnosis shows in the UK. So a good deal of stage work has migrated to foreign holiday resorts, for now.

Good riddance say some, but I think it is actually time for the evolution of a completely different kind of hypnosis presentation that educates the audience, as well as astonishing them and being good family entertainment. It is time for the notion of the hypnotist as a person with 'special powers' to be de-bunked, and for hypnosis to be properly understood by everyone, and that must include understanding the old stage hypnosis shows that have done so much to shape people's general misconception of hypnosis in the past.

Whatever the word 'hypnosis' means to you, unless you have studied hypnotherapy in detail and have a good deal of personal experience with it – or read the first volume of this book already - you will have no accurate understanding of my profession, or how hypnotherapy works. In fact, you will probably have a very inaccurate notion of what we therapists actually do with hypnosis, and may imagine it to be similar to what a stage hypnotist apparently does. This is because most people have never even seen any hypnotherapy, let alone experienced it for themselves. What they have actually seen is stage hypnosis, and so their general impression of what hypnosis is will be largely based on what they *think* they see in stage hypnosis. We might add to that the general impressions they have gleaned from anything they have ever read about hypnotism in a newspaper, heard somebody say, or maybe saw in a movie that referred to hypnosis in some way. Those things will usually have been written or said by someone who really knows nothing about hypnosis, but has seen a stage demonstration somewhere.

We advise one another: "Don't believe everything you read"... and everyone agrees this is wise. Most people believe what they see though. Think how often you have heard someone say: "I wouldn't have believed it myself, but I saw it with my own eyes!" as if what *really* happened must be the same as what *apparently* happened. Yet we all know, from enjoying many skilled performances of 'magic' on stage and television, that there can be a huge difference between the real and the apparent, and that the eyes can very easily be deceived. The key difference is that when a modern audience is watching an illusionist perform they already know it is an illusion before it begins, so they can only be amazed by how good the illusion looks. They know for sure the woman has not really been sawn in half, or whatever. It is the *artistry,* the skill of the illusionist they are appreciating, if anything. Nobody runs for the exit in terror as the saw-blade apparently cuts deep into the box.

Yet there must have been a time when people did. Modern 'magic' shows have their origins in ruses used in ancient religious or witchcraft ceremonies designed to terrify, or otherwise convince and impress the ignorant. Various aspects of modern stage hypnosis also have their roots in this but of course, these ruses are only convincing if you do not know how they are done. Once they are properly explained, everybody just says: "Oh, so that's how they do it", and that is the end of that. Clever perhaps, but certainly not mysterious or alarming any more. Perfectly understandable in fact, without any 'special powers' actually being involved at all. The ignorance of the audience, then, is always a crucial factor if they are going to be amazed. They must not know how it's done.

Stage hypnosis has a history, and it is a very long one. Even in its modern form, rowdy stage antics involving willing members of the audience go back well over a century in this part of the world. Such shows were quite popular in Victorian times, as were all sorts of other 'mysterious' and 'amazing' things, all of which *suggested* the demonstration of super-normal powers. There was escapology, there were amazing mind-reading acts, mediums and séances, and of course the ever-popular illusionists we still see today. Stage hypnosis developed its modern form – with audience participation as its central convincer – amid this wave of spectacular live theatre performances where the aim was to amaze, and which were probably the best form of entertainment available at the time.

As the decades have passed, most of these types of acts have had their cover blown, so to speak, so that everybody now knows they are illusions and some have pretty much disappeared from the world of entertainment as a result. Those that remain are now openly acknowledged as illusions, like stage magic. Stage hypnosis is the only exception.

## The Beyond

Mediums and the paranormal generally have remained popular within the culture at large, but more as an alternative belief-system than a form of entertainment usually. Uri Geller, who created an enormous stir in the 1970s when he first became internationally famous, seems to have been the last example of the (apparently) paranormal performer actively seeking the spotlight 'to convince the world', as it were. Today's media circus - cynical, ruthless, irreverent and very quickly bored – seems a hostile environment for people genuinely interested and involved in studying the paranormal. Even when these subjects do come up in the media, which they always will because they capture the imagination, they are usually edited and presented with a less-than-serious touch, as if such subjects are slightly beneath the medium really. (I mean the broadcast medium of course, not the Doris Stokes variety.)

Hypnotherapy is not remotely anything to do with the paranormal, but is often treated by journalists and media people generally in a similar sort of way, which is one of the reasons most hypnotherapists tend to avoid the media, leaving them only stage hypnotists to muck about with. Also stage hypnosis lends itself better to the fairly impatient, instant impact nature of most media production. Programme makers and producers prefer to suppose all hypnosis is like stage hypnosis, and aren't interested in learning about any realities that might turn out to require more time and production costs to truly understand and demonstrate to the public.

The old Reithian ideal - that broadcasting exists partly to educate us - has struggled to survive at all even at the BBC, largely because of increasing competition for the viewers' attention. The early ambitions of some television companies particularly – such as the moral outlook of Sydney Bernstein at Granada Television in Manchester - are sadly a thing of the past. It would be a rare TV producer nowadays who might seriously aim to investigate hypnotherapy in depth. Even one-off specials are rare, and often feature a narrative and editorial handling that makes real experts in hypnotherapy want to shoot the television, Elvis-style. There is rarely any real understanding coming across and most TV producers would probably assume their listeners and viewers might care little for such understanding anyway but prefer to consume a recognisable snapshot of their existing general impressions – even if those are wrong.

## Strangely Unchanged

Of all the old 'Amazing Powers' types of stage performance, only Stage Hypnosis remains pretty much as it was a century ago, with its central illusion largely intact: the suggestion that the hypnotist has 'power' and can literally control the mind or behaviour of another person. Many people are still convinced this is actually true, despite the obvious fact that if stage hypnotists could really control the minds of others they would rule the world, not be doing summer season end-of-the-pier shows in Blackpool. The fact that you only ever see this 'mind control' performance on stage or screen gives it away - it is a piece of entertainment. And like many things in the world of entertainment, it is not what it appears to be. But it helps to have a bit of inside knowledge if you want to understand what is really going on.

Without inside information to explain the performance, members of the audience really only have two possible conclusions open to them: either it is a complete fraud and all these people are in on the act, or else the stage hypnotist is a man of amazing powers over other people's minds. If neither of those options convinces you completely – and they shouldn't, because they are both untrue – then you are left feeling confused and not really knowing what to think.

The truth is actually somewhere in the middle, and has a lot more to do with ordinary human psychology than it has to do with anything mysterious. In fact there is a series of illusions involved. Like all illusions, these can be quite convincing provided the spectator does not know how they actually work. The audience 'see it with their own eyes' but what they are 'seeing' is the illusion. "Seeing is believing" as they say, but reality can be something else entirely - so I shall explain the reality in specific detail as we proceed.

Another notable group of performers, modern-day healers and evangelists, when they are working with a credulous crowd also use techniques and suggestions that experienced hypnotists recognize immediately. But whether they are using them knowingly and cynically is another matter. Some of them probably are, but it is also perfectly possible to copy a performance that has impressed or 'inspired' you, without understanding how it really works, and yet genuinely believe that the amazing effects on others are caused by some other factor: God, angels, spirits, the devil – whatever.

Even stage hypnotists themselves do not all truly understand the dynamics involved in their own shows, they just know how to do it. Many of them have simply learned a routine, and then they perform it. All it takes is the quick-wittedness of the natural stage performer, and some brass neck. I have discussed hypnosis with stage performers who turned out to have little or no real understanding of what is actually happening – and why should they? You don't have to know how a car works to drive one perfectly well, and unless you take the trouble and time to learn all the intricate details – and many drivers can't be bothered – then you are no car expert. Few *stage* hypnotists are experts in how the human mind really functions, or why stage hypnosis produces the effects it does. There are some exceptions of course, but they are certainly not going to explain it to their audience. That would spoil everything!

Yes, stage hypnosis is really just a series of illusions aimed at the audience, it's just that most members of the audience don't realise that. Or even if they suspect something, they don't know the details because the stage hypnotist is never going to explain anything. This is because he doesn't want his audience to *understand* hypnosis, far from it. The stage hypnotist is setting out to sell an idea to the audience - an idea which is false in the first place. The idea is that he (and it is always a 'he' - you never see a woman doing this) has power or influence over the minds of other people. In reality he has no such power but he is going to make it look as if he does, and so long as the audience does not know quite how that works - and they don't - it can look quite convincing on the face of it.

The stage hypnotist sets out to convince the audience by the end of the show that there is a mysterious state of mind called "hypnosis", and that this is some strange state of mind quite outside of the audiences' normal mental experience. This fanciful notion then extends to encourage the impression that if the hypnotist can get an audience member "into hypnosis", or "under", then that person will do anything the hypnotist says, no matter how ridiculous it is. These are the general ideas stage hypnotism aims to convey... and if that is your personal impression about hypnosis, then the stage hypnosis demonstrations you have seen in the past have been pretty successful in getting those false ideas across to you. Either that or you have simply picked up this impression from other people anyway, who did not realize that their vague ideas about hypnosis were wrong.

So, let's get this firmly established now: the idea that the hypnotist is controlling other people is simply what the stage hypnotist wants you to think. Some of them may even partly believe it themselves, because they may not have any more real insight regarding the participants' behaviour than their audience, they have just learned through experience that not everybody will respond – a fact they hope the audience will overlook, because it does rather detract from the suggestion that the hypnotist has power!

As a direct result of the existence of Stage Hypnosis - and the fact that everybody has seen an example of it somewhere, but probably never seen any hypnotherapy - I have to explain all of this in detail to every one of my new clients before I can start working with them. Before I can even begin to explain what hypnosis actually is, I have to spend about ten or fifteen minutes explaining what it isn't. This is most important because if I don't bother, and leave my clients with their original notions of what hypnosis is, they have half as much chance of rapid success, if that. Any hypnotherapist who does not clear their client's misconceptions of hypnosis effectively will be nowhere near as successful as they otherwise would be.

Hypnosis, you see, is not 'mind control' by somebody else. It is not brainwashing and it is not a mystery at all, once it is properly explained. Anyone who reads the whole of this book with genuine interest will have a pretty good understanding of the subject by the end of it. And although the human mind seems to be endlessly fascinating, as does human behaviour, *hypnosis* can be effectively mastered far more easily as a subject, especially once you have fully understood all the things that it is not, and let go of the fantasy version.

Hypnotherapy is certainly not something somebody 'does to you', although most people think it is. Even the idea that hypnotists 'hypnotize' people is actually rather misleading, although of course two people can certainly participate in a rigmarole that looks very much like that. Before we can become truly expert in the subject, first we have to lay the stage hypnosis ghost, because this daft spectre has been haunting hypnotherapists for well over a hundred years. And really it is only an illusion, which plays on the fears and ignorance of people who do not realize it is just an illusion.

N.B.: In calling it an illusion, I do not mean that hypnosis does not exist but that the whole show is designed to suggest to the audience that the hypnotist is controlling the mind of the person in hypnosis, and that they are therefore effectively in his power. In reality, their behaviour is not controlled by the hypnotist but by their own Subconscious mind, which normally controls a good deal of our behaviour anyway, as I demonstrate with numerous ordinary examples throughout this book. On the stage, the participant's Subconscious mind certainly does not have to respond to any of the Stage Hypnotist's suggestions, it has a choice. And indeed many people wouldn't, however deep in trance they were because they would have no personal motivation to accept those particular suggestions. That is why *those* people are never on the stage, or never on the stage for long. The illusion is really about the real role of the hypnotist himself, and this false impression of what he is actually doing is cleverly suggested to the audience throughout the show - through the hypnotist's behaviour and the language he uses deliberately in order to mislead the audience.

In order to create this imaginary world of mind-control on the stage, the stage hypnotist needs some little helpers and he gets them from the audience. It is this selection process that is really the key to the whole stage performance – who gets to be on the stage, and why them - because he has to get this right, or this is never going to be convincing. When these performances are shown on TV, this selection part is nearly always edited out, so the TV audience viewing at home doesn't see it at all. If you go along to a live stage hypnosis performance, you will see the selection process take place but it is carefully disguised to look like a random selection. In reality, it is a careful selection of the right sort of person. It is not exactly a fraud because these people are not plants or stooges - they are real members of the audience. But it is not a random selection. These individuals are being carefully chosen, according to personality type and attitude on the night.

Who does he want on the stage? The kind of people who want to be in a stage hypnosis show, that's who! And that rules out most of the audience straight away, because they certainly do not. When people go along to see one of these performances, most of them are going to watch: they don't want to be starring in it themselves. The majority prefer to let someone else take to the stage and be in the spotlight. But in any sizeable crowd there will be some ideal candidates – who may not even realize that they are ideal candidates, but the hypnotist knows how to locate them.

Now the main difference between these people and everyone else is simple, and it has nothing to do with how hypnotizable they are, or suggestible or susceptible. That word 'susceptible' irritates me, because more often than not the word is being used by people who imagine that they would probably be *unsusceptible* themselves because they assume that anyone who responds to any kind of hypnosis is in some way weak or easily-led, whereas in fact the people using that word are just ignorant. They are wrong on all counts. A response to any hypnotic procedure indicates only one thing: an inclination to respond. A lack of response indicates either a fear of participating, unwillingness to participate, stupidity to a really uncommon degree or a complete lack of imagination and/or emotional drive. Usually it is a simple unwillingness to participate. Sometimes this is termed 'resistance' but I think that word is a bit dramatic – they just don't feel inclined to respond.

Most people just do not wish to be on a stage in the first place, not for any reason, if they can possibly avoid it. They prefer not to be the centre of attention, because they are afraid of making a fool of themselves in front of all these people. We are talking about the majority of the audience: most people feel this way because they are not attention-seekers. So if the stage hypnotist were to take someone like that and put them in the spotlight, he would only make them painfully self-conscious and anxious to return to their seat. People who feel that way about being the centre of attention are not much use for entertainment purposes, are they? He doesn't want anyone like that on the stage - he wants them in the audience where they belong. But he doesn't want them to understand that because he wants those same people to imagine, all the way through the show: "If he could get me up there, he could make me do all those bizarre things, with the mysterious power of hypnosis!" Which is not the case at all.

The type of people the stage hypnotist is more interested in have a completely different feeling about the idea of being centre-stage. Some people *love* to be the centre of attention, and in any audience there will always be a handful of them who will do any daft thing you like if it means they can hog the spotlight for a while and get some applause. Very often these people do not have any talent, to speak of – in fact, these are the best type because they never normally get invited onto a stage and rarely have much of an audience, which means they will probably jump at the chance if they get one. They are frustrated performers... and you only have to look at karaoke to realize how many people we are talking about here, there are quite a lot of them around.

Now karaoke is a slightly different matter, and some of the people who get up and do their bit can actually sing to some extent. I'm sure you will have noticed, though, that quite a few of these amateur vocalists can't sing a note, yet this sad fact does not put them off. One or two of them might be quite deluded about this, but most of them *know* they do not have any real talent. They don't let that hold them back at all though because they are not murdering that song for the audience's sake in the first place. They are simply performing for their own enjoyment. Really they are acting out the fantasy of being an entertainer - which they would love to be, but they're not. Karaoke offers them an opportunity to *play* at being an entertainer, not just with a hairbrush in front of their bedroom mirror but with a real microphone, a real audience and maybe even real applause. For anyone who is not too shy, this can be genuinely appealing and may indeed be their only opportunity ever to perform. And this has now become a socially-acceptable form of entertainment in its own right. Apparently.

## A Little Aside, about How Wrong We Can Be

Many years ago my eldest brother Martin was teaching English in Japan. He lived there for two years, and being a linguist, he took the opportunity to learn to speak Japanese. Shortly after he returned to the U.K. we were visited by a group of Japanese people with whom he had been working, and we all went out for a meal. The cultural differences between the Japanese and the English – well, the Japanese and *anyone,* really – are so great that this would have been a surreal enough experience without the marvellous, yet slightly disturbing sound of my own brother speaking fluent Japanese. It was probably only disturbing because my only previous experience of people speaking Japanese was in films like *Bridge Over The River Kwai.* I had to battle a mad urge to resort to childish sibling mimicry: "Ah so! Martin-san, how it feel to be back in U.K.?"

During the two years he was in Japan, Martin sent me letters telling me all about how different life was in that part of the world and we both found some of these things quite amusing, such as the fact that no-one in Japan would cross the road in an impromptu fashion, they would only cross at the pedestrian crossings... and that there were street vending machines that sold bottles of whisky. We felt pretty certain that if someone put one of those in a street in any British city they would never get the chance to re-stock it because it simply wouldn't be there when they returned. But most astonishing of all, I thought, was the letter I received which described the bizarre Japanese practice of handing a microphone to anyone in a bar and letting them sing one of their favourite songs to a backing track, regardless of whether they could sing or not! I shook my head in disbelief at the baffling madness of Japanese culture, knowing for sure that such a thing could never become popular in the country I grew up in. Within a year of that it was here.

I now suspect that when people die off naturally, it is not really old age that kills them. I think it is just that after seven or eight decades of surprising changes they simply cannot take any more unexpected developments and can't escape the feeling that they don't really belong here anymore. I'm only in my late forties, but I'm starting to feel like that already.

# Back Onstage

People divide up into two sorts: spectators and performers. There are many more spectators than performers, but some of the performers have never developed a talent or an outlet for it, so they have little opportunity to get into the spotlight. Therefore they are usually limited to amateur dramatics, or more commonly karaoke, stage hypnosis and those occasional TV opportunities like The X-Factor, Pop Idol or Big Brother.

People like this may appear outwardly confident in ordinary social situations, or they may not. Some are obviously attention-seekers in every situation, but others may be quiet or even shy in normal situations, yet feel drawn to the stage or the spotlight. Some actors also find liberation in assuming a role on the stage or in front of the cameras, and become bolder than they are in ordinary life. It is really the opposite of what happens to spectators when the spotlight turns upon them. Performers may not always be obvious performers, but they find being in the limelight thrilling. The real world vanishes, and the magical world of theatre or television replaces it. They are immediately entranced, and the conscious mind – which normally inhibits their attention-seeking behaviour – is no longer in the driving seat. There is no mental stress, but there is adrenaline, and although they may be hesitant at first, once the first gale of laughter or round of applause hits them, they are off and running. They are accepted in this new role, and it is so much more fun than any role they have played before. They are a hit. They are a star! Now you would have to drag them off with a hook if you want to get them out of that spotlight.

When performers without any specific talent go along to a stage hypnosis show, they know this is one of the rare occasions when ordinary people can get to star in a show, and win some applause. Some are rather hoping it is going to be them, because they know they will have more fun *doing that* than watching somebody else get to be the centre of attention all evening. These people usually tend to be competitive for attention, and have less fear of making fools of themselves. They are quite happy to be part of a spectacle if it makes everybody laugh. But some don't realise consciously they are going to feel that way until they actually find themselves in the spotlight, because they may never have had that experience before. They may be quite pleasantly surprised to discover that, for them, the whole thing is quite a buzz. Suddenly they are an entertainer, happy to be applauded for bursting into song, happy to be applauded for clowning around or just following ridiculous instructions. They know they don't have to, but as long as they are getting applause and putting smiles on faces, well... that's entertainment, isn't it?

So all the stage hypnotist needs to do at the start of the show is find these people and get them on the stage, but preferably make it look like a random selection, so the rest of the audience never recognise that these people are significantly different from them. The 'players' really select themselves because their desire to participate overrides their conscious doubts about the whole thing. Once they are part of the show, the conscious hesitations will quickly evaporate if everything goes okay for them, and they can lose themselves in the action. They are playing a role, after all – the role of the hypnotised person in a hypnosis show. This is essentially why they then behave in a way the majority of the audience cannot relate to. It isn't because they are 'under hypnosis', or indeed under the control of someone else. It is because they suddenly feel free to express themselves without inhibition in this magical setting. It is an opportunity to let the natural-born entertainer in them come out and play for a while.

Now I'm not suggesting that everyone who ever took part in a stage hypnosis performance was exactly this sort of person, but I would say that everyone who was *more than happy* to take part in a stage hypnosis performance, enjoyed the experience, and would happily do it again, was exactly this sort of person. There are even people who volunteer themselves with the conscious intention of de-bunking the whole business of hypnosis, only to find themselves pointing at UFOs in the sky or doing an Elvis impression, and afterwards their conscious mind might be quite confused about that. But it's easy enough to understand once you learn about the nature of the Subconscious mind. The Subconscious knew nothing of those conscious intentions but seized the opportunity to be Elvis for five minutes. "I'm the King of Rock and Roll! There's my audience, they love me!" Go for it.

In the Subconscious mind, the imagination reigns supreme. How do you think Elvis invented *himself?* There is a very fine line between genius and ridiculous, and much as I appreciate Elvis at his best, he certainly crossed the line in both directions at various times during his amazing career. We could all behave like that really. The only difference between us is how we personally react to the experience of being the centre of attention, or finding ourselves suddenly in the spotlight. And of course I am only talking about the business of performing here, not talent. Elvis Presley's recording success had far more to do with his unique vocal talent than his stage act, which wouldn't have got him very far if he hadn't been much of a singer.

This is what TV programmes like the X-Factor and Pop Idol are demonstrating over and over again. The vast majority of the population are spectators, and don't want to join in with that game but might enjoy watching it. Thousands apply for a chance to play the game, and most of them are performers by nature even if they have zero talent. A small percentage have enough talent to get them through to the later rounds, but only one or two end up with a recording contract and even then they have to work very hard to turn that into a career. In contrast, the vast majority of the thousands who applied to play the game in the first place could be the star of a stage hypnosis show.

True performers love the whole thing, don't really want it to end, and really don't mind afterwards how carried away they got. They enjoy being the centre of attention and think it is all good harmless fun, both during and after the show. Experienced stage hypnotists will home in on this sort of character and leave everyone else alone, because performers understand the deal, especially if they have done things like this before. Even if they haven't, they soon find that the more they put on a performance, the more the audience seem to like them and the more of a buzz they get out of it. So even if they don't have any particular talent, they can still play the role of the entertainer in this type of performance, and discover for themselves that there is no business like show business.

In practice, it is quite easy for the stage hypnotist to locate suitable candidates at the start of the show because these are the only people who want to be found, or betray any inclination to come and play. The rest of the crowd have no intention of joining in, and it shows. Imagine you are the stage hypnotist. As you approach your audience looking for volunteers for your stage hypnosis show, the people who see you coming towards them react. Most of them instinctively shy away, trying not to catch your eye. These people have DON'T PICK ME written all over them, they emphatically do not want to play, they only want to be entertained. Some make a big show of shying away, but they are over-reacting and do want to play: body-language experts (hypnotists usually are) will easily spot the difference. A few people have an eager, rapt facial expression that more or less begs PICK ME! and they never take their eyes off the hypnotist. Through this body language they promise to follow all instructions to the letter because they want to be the star of the show so much that it hurts.

There are lots of ways for the stage hypnotist to go about selecting his candidates. He could just walk through the crowd and select individuals, which looks impressive because the people in the audience don't realise that they are unconsciously signalling willingness or unwillingness as he approaches them. So this method looks like a random selection – creating the misleading suggestion that he can put absolutely anyone in his show - or else makes it seem as if he is psychic, effortlessly zeroing in on his people, as if he knows more about them than they do. The relief of those who are *not* picked is palpable, but they needn't have worried. They were never going to be picked. They don't want to play. The hypnotist can see that. In fact it was blindingly obvious, from the way they reacted as he came near. Even if they did nothing at all, they were clearly signalling to him that they were not giving away any clues... in other words they were not going to help him at all with his show here tonight.

Another very common method of sorting the sheep from the goats - the sheep are the audience by the way, it is the participants who will be acting the goat - is to invite the whole audience to play a game. This also serves to distract the audience from the fact that people are being selected here, not picked at random. The audience will be intrigued by the game whether they play it or not, and simply by being intrigued they are a little more open to suggestion than a person who is not intrigued (i.e. not interested in the least). Don't forget that it is not only the people who end up on the stage who are the target of the stage hypnotist's suggestions, but the whole audience. He is selling you a fantasy, the imaginary notion that one person can control the behaviour of several others, via some mysterious power – the 'Power of Hypnosis'.

Probably the most commonly-used game is the hand-clasp, in which everyone is invited to clasp their hands together tightly and "concentrate on them" (actually nothing to do with the effort of conscious concentration, this is fixation of the gaze, it is a trance induction), using the power of their mind to *imagine* them becoming stuck, as if glued together. Then as if stuck together by superglue, so that you couldn't pull them apart even if you tried. Then to imagine that they are not real hands at all, but a perfect sculpture, carved from a solid block of wood and are one solid mass... not really separate at all, but joined permanently together. Now cast in bronze... a solid heavy mass that obviously could never, ever be pulled apart by human effort... now when I tell you to, and not before...on the count of three, try to pull your hands apart *and find that you can't!* One! Two! THREE! You can't pull them apart, you can't! Really, really try! Try harder! In fact the harder you try, the more those hands seem completely unmovable, however hard you try, you cannot pull them apart!

Now if you have never been invited to participate in such a game under those live, theatrical conditions you may be utterly convinced, on a conscious level, that you would not find any difficulty separating your hands. You may be quite certain, on a conscious level, that your hands are under your own control not the control of the hypnotist. And you would certainly be right about that because that is true of everybody in the audience. The hypnotist knows that too - that is, if he truly understands how this works. Some stage hypnotists don't really understand it, they just know that it does work. But if you think your hands are under your *conscious* control all the time, just because you are *able* to consciously control them under ordinary circumstances... well, that is where you would be wrong. But that doesn't mean the hypnotist can control them. Nor does it mean that you would necessarily respond to his suggestion and find it impossible to part your hands. It rather depends upon how you *feel* about the whole idea in the first place, and the implications of responding.

If you present an audience with the opportunity to play a game like this you are going to get a range of different reactions, because you are talking to lots of different people. Some will not play the game, either because they just don't like joining in with any kind of audience participation, or because they are afraid of what will happen if they do play – will they end up on the stage? Remember, most audience members do not want to play any role in the show, so any that are really afraid of risking that may not play at all. Some people even sit on their hands, to make damn sure they don't get stuck together. Actually there was no danger of them being selected – they were simply unaware of that fact. Some of the ones who don't play the handclasp game are simply afraid of hypnosis itself because they don't understand it. It is a simple fear of the 'unknown'.

All the people covered by the paragraph above regarded the suggestion to play the hand-clasp game as an unwelcome suggestion, for one reason or another. The suggestion did not appeal to them, and the first time we are presented with an unwelcome suggestion, we are not likely to accept it. For some people though it is not the suggestion to play the game that is unwelcome, they don't mind that. It is the suggestion that their hands will become stuck fast: that is the bit they regard as unwelcome. So they accept the suggestion to play the game, but reject all the suggestions about their hands, because they do not want that to happen. We only accept the suggestions we find acceptable, all other suggestions are ignored or rejected. Fear may be the reason they do not like the sound of being unable to separate their hands. Fear of hypnosis, fear of loss of control or fear of ending up on the stage. If this is the dominant emotion, the Subconscious uses this as the yardstick to measure how they feel about that suggestion, overall – and does nothing with it.

Some people who reject the handclasp suggestions are not really afraid, but they are reading the suggestion a different way - they regard it as *an attempt by the hypnotist to stick their hands together,* and if they regard that as a challenge to their authority over their own body, well again, this is a 'control' issue, but more a case of determination to retain complete autonomy rather than allow the hypnotist to call the shots, where their own actions are concerned. So it may not be *fear* of loss of control in every case, but sometimes just a straight preference. The idea of someone else influencing their behaviour or even thought-patterns just doesn't appeal to that individual. So they might play - or go through the motions of playing - but they have no *desire* to respond, so they don't.

## The Erroneous Assumptions of the Unresponsive

These people who do not respond to the suggestions above may be under the impression that the people who do respond are somehow different from them. They imagine that those other people are 'more susceptible', 'more suggestible', or maybe just 'easily influenced'. Perhaps they are just 'weak-minded' or 'easily led'... or just do as they are told generally. Possibly those people are imagining the whole thing, even putting it on perhaps, simply pretending to respond? These are the possibilities that may run through the non-respondent's mind.

On the whole, though, people who did not find the suggestion appealing on any level and therefore did not respond will be happy with their non-response - obviously, because they got what they wanted. Some of them may even feel a bit superior to the people who apparently cannot separate their hands. "Those people seem unable to resist the will of the hypnotist," they tell themselves, "whereas I cannot be hypnotized, my mind is too strong!" So says their conscious mind, which will be absolutely convinced that *it* was in control the whole time. And certainly, the conscious mind usually does reject the suggestion, mainly because the conscious mind did not believe the response was even possible. But in reality, this conscious opinion is common to everyone the first time they play the game, including the ones who *do* respond. Hence their genuine amazement when they cannot part their hands.

In the persons who did not respond, however, their conscious rejection of the suggestion and general disbelief is not the *real* reason the response didn't happen, although they will think it is. It is entirely because their Subconscious rejected it too. You see, responding to suggestions of this sort - or not responding - has nothing to do with your conscious beliefs, intentions or expectations. It is entirely an emotional matter: how much *desire* there is to respond, and how much *fear* is contesting it. The Subconscious weighs it in the balance, finds in favour of one or the other and then it either responds or it doesn't according to the apparent preference. The conscious mind has nothing to do with it, but of course the conscious mind will only come to realize that if the Subconscious does choose to respond. A lack of Subconscious response allows the conscious mind to continue to believe it makes all the decisions about behaviour simply because the lack of response happens to coincide with the conscious expectation. But the conscious mind is completely thrown when the Subconscious *does* respond, because it genuinely did not expect that to happen and there is no conscious understanding of why it did. The stage hypnotist certainly isn't going to try to explain it, whether he understands it himself or not.

Now, because the hypnotist suggested that would happen, and much to their conscious amazement it did, the people who cannot part their hands may well conclude that the hypnotist caused it to happen, by some mysterious 'power' that is outside their own control. This is an illusion, because their own Subconscious responses are not outside their control at all - merely outside their conscious control - and there are many ordinary examples of that as I demonstrated elsewhere when explaining compulsive habits. Still, most of the people who did respond will be quite happy with the surprising fact that they apparently cannot part their hands with a conscious effort, because of course they got what they *wanted*, even if it was not quite what they expected. When you expect little, and much to your surprise you get success, the common response is delight.

Notice how this has absolutely nothing to do with how 'hypnotizable' or 'suggestible' anybody is, but *how much they want to play,* for their own reasons. All that hypnosis business is nowhere near as important for the stage hypnotist as the question of who wants to play. (Likewise for the hypnotherapist, hypnotism is nowhere near as important as how much the client wants to change.) Still, the stage hypnotist wants the audience to think hypnosis is important because he needs to build up their impression of his own role in the affair far beyond what it actually is, and the whole point of a game like this is to create the impression that something wild and crazy is beginning to happen and that the hypnotist is making it happen! In truth it is all perfectly understandable once you learn how the mind really works.

Now at this point the stage hypnotist will invite all the people with their hands stuck together to come up on stage... but that is a different suggestion again, and some of the people who were quite happy to play the game, and quite happy to respond to the game, may have a good deal less enthusiasm about being on the stage, so they may reject the third suggestion and stay where they are. This proves that any suggestion can be rejected at any time, regardless of any previous co-operation, if there is reluctance concerning that particular idea. These people are never 'in the power' of the hypnotist - as the show strongly suggests - even if they have the confused impression that they must be. All their responses, positive or negative, are consistent with the sum of their Subconscious desires tempered by the extent of any fears, and it is their Subconscious mind, not the hypnotist, which directs their response. The hypnotist can only aim suggestions at their Subconscious mind. He can never direct their Subconscious *response*.

This is the variable factor that makes some people assume that hypnosis does not 'work on' some people. Whether a person responds at that given moment or not largely depends upon what they feel like doing. The twist is, your Subconscious mind may spontaneously feel like doing something your conscious mind may be disinterested in, such as behaving as if you are James Bond whenever the James Bond theme tune is played, for example (a common stage hypnosis suggestion). Your conscious mind may think that sounds like a silly idea. Ridiculous, actually. Unbeknown to your conscious mind, though, your Subconscious may already be muttering to itself: "Vodka martini – shaken, not stirred." What man never fantasized about being someone like James Bond? Apart from those who fantasized about being *with* him, I mean. The Subconscious mind of most men would love the idea of being the world's greatest secret agent - effortless seducer of women, licensed to kill! And drive like a maniac. Just like the karaoke singer who loves the idea of being Gloria Gaynor. We do have fantasy lives you know.

The hypnotist is controlling none of this. He is merely taking advantage of the law of averages. Most men in the audience would secretly love to be just like James Bond, but of course many will inhibit their response to one or other of these introductory, 'selection' suggestions for some reason. Yet in any sizeable audience there are always going to be a few people who turn out to have no fear of playing any of these games and find the whole thing exciting, not daunting. So if they also find the prospect of being centre-stage appealing and crave audience approval, and applause, they might well respond - and then go on responding just as long as it feels good, encouraged by the hypnotist to some degree but mainly encouraged by the laughter and applause, which can be intoxicating. Once you have got to this level of excitement, why inhibit anything? This individual is now bathed in mass approval, probably more approval than they have ever known previously – why stop now?

That's the way the Subconscious is looking at it. Don't forget, the Subconscious knows this is all a game within an entertainment context. It's just having fun here, and the audience seems to like it so where's the harm? The hypnotist is simply directing suggestions at the performer. He is not directing their behaviour - it is their own Subconscious mind controlling that. This is not really "The Power of Suggestion" because there is no power in a suggestion itself, which is exactly why some people do not react. It is how you feel about that suggestion - right there and then - which governs any response. It is really *the power of the imagination, driven by Subconscious desire and uninhibited by any other factor* that we really see playing itself out in some people. The power of suggestion sounds snappier of course, but is misleading really.

No, the hypnotist cannot direct the person's Subconscious response, he can only direct various suggestions at them and hope he picked the right punter. What may make his little helper quite confused, on a conscious level, is the fact that they may well be aware that their conscious mind is not directing all this crazy behaviour either – and the conscious mind may be rather puzzled by that, because it is accustomed to the notion that it directs all decisions and behaviour.

This is the factor that baffles the participants on a conscious level, and also those people in the audience who know them well.

Most people do not even realize they *have* a Subconscious mind, they certainly do not know what it does or how differently it sees the world from the way the conscious mind looks at it. So when the performers in a stage hypnosis show are getting more and more carried away as the evening progresses, it is not surprising that people in the audience who know them personally may regard their behaviour as out of character, as if something very strange has happened to them. Their antics on the stage may well be very different from their usual behaviour but that is really because they do not usually have permission to adopt the persona of James Bond. If they did that in everyday life they certainly wouldn't get a huge round of applause. The behaviour is dramatically different because the circumstances are different, and indeed this may be a unique experience for them, the first time they have ever been 'the star of the show' and going down a storm. How often does this side of their personality get a chance to shine?

## The Second Selection Process

Not all of the people who originally make their way to the stage in response to the hypnotist's invitation are quite what he is looking for. Some will be weeded out, told "thank you for playing", and sent back to their seats, usually without any explanation. Anyone whose attention is wandering - waving to their mates in the audience or looking around rather than paying close attention, any jokers who look a bit too cocky - these are some of the people the show doesn't need. Remember, the hypnotist has no power over anyone. Those who may have gone up there to mess about or make a monkey of the hypnotist will not be allowed to play at all, because it would be easy for them to do that and it would just spoil the show. It is the people who are happy to play the correct role who will be allowed to stay in the spotlight, and that is both their motivation and their reward.

Once these people have selected themselves and are up on the stage, they know they are now regarded by the audience as 'the hypnotist's chosen ones', and so they are expected to take part in the show. This adds another level of subtle suggestion. They know instinctively that if they play the game properly it will entertain and please the audience, whereas if they back out or sabotage the proceedings then the audience will feel a bit let down. Therefore they are likely to feel under some obligation, having allowed themselves to progress thus far, to rise to the occasion. They know what they are in for anyway, because they have seen it all before on TV. It's just a lot of daft larking about to entertain people. It certainly isn't difficult and they don't have to learn the part like an actor would because the hypnotist gives them suggestions and cues all the way along. If they act out the suggestions they get to be a star for an hour or so. It's as easy as that.

## Settling In

At the beginning of the show, a good stage hypnotist will be very reassuring and not demand anything much from the players, just make them feel welcome and relieve the tension with general banter that helps everyone to feel comfortable in their role. It is also useful, during this 'getting to know you' introductory bit, to ask participants a few innocuous questions to which the answer is very likely to be "yes", such as "Are you alright?", "Are you here with friends?" "Where do you live/Do you like living there?" "Are you having a good night?" These questions help to get them talking and build a little confidence but their main purpose is to get them used to saying "yes" to the hypnotist. Once they have said "yes" several times and they are still apparently safe and secure, this gives their Subconscious mind the initial impression that the hypnotist is in charge and can be trusted, so it will probably be OK if we follow the hypnotist's lead. Don't forget, most of these people are not accustomed to being on a stage, so in addition to feeling excited are also feeling a bit vulnerable. The hypnotist does this sort of thing for a living, so he is the expert up here on the stage, they need him onside. Stick with the leader, that's the safe thing to do. Don't upset him, and don't try to get too clever. It is the hypnotist's show after all, it's not the volunteer's show and the only excuse they have for being up here in the limelight is to play their role in his show. And they already know what that is, because they have seen this sort of thing before on the TV. All they have to do is follow the leader, and they should soon be enjoying applause and laughter.

In for a penny, in for a pound - that is the emotional position of the participants at this point. So the hypnotist knows that if he handles them carefully to begin with, until the audience's later approval and applause kicks in and makes them bolder in due course, they should be with him all the way.

Now, stage hypnotists vary a little as to how they put a show together. Some will take their chosen people backstage at the start and 'prep' them. This mainly consists of making them familiar with various words and signals so they will easily recognize them at any time in the show. This hidden procedure adds to the mystery from the audience's point of view, but also creates a delay that detracts from a really slick performance.

The more confident performers are unlikely to bother with this, and it is partly their confidence that makes it unnecessary. They know they can rely on all the notions and expectations that already exist in the minds of their volunteers - plus the fact that these people clearly wish to be involved in the performance - to produce all the right responses at the right moments. And they usually will, but the most confident performers of all will realise that it doesn't even matter if anything goes wrong because in a live performance audiences love the bits that apparently don't go according to plan, and stage hypnosis shows are meant to seem like pretty anarchic affairs anyway.

True spontaneity will include unplanned deviations from direction, and these add a bit of edge: an unpredictability that also serves to convince the audience that the other bits that worked perfectly were not rehearsed, but were genuine spontaneity too. As long as the hypnotist doesn't seem to mind if something 'goes wrong', then the audience certainly won't mind. In fact they will probably admire him more for remaining confident and good-humoured whether things go right or not. He cannot lose in fact, as long as he is confident in himself. He is surrounded by entertainers just waiting for suggestions for how to make themselves more popular.

So the people who end up on the stage are happy to be there, feel inclined to stay and have a preference to win the approval of the hypnotist and the audience. They understand instinctively that this will require a performance, which they know they can produce. The more enthusiastic the performance is, the more approval they will win. The people who make up the final group – traditionally called "the committee" – are therefore not going to mess up the hypnotist's show. They want to be in it, and don't want to disappoint anyone because they now have an opportunity to be one of the stars of the show. They know that the hypnotist who has allowed them this opportunity can either help them to succeed in that, or take the chance away from them if their response to the suggestions is disappointing. Their every inclination is to please him - to be *safe* (following their natural instinct for self-preservation because they feel pretty exposed up here in the spotlight) and also to be *successful* (their personal desire to seek approval and applause).

Spectators often refer later to the ridiculous things that the stage hypnotist 'made' people do, but in reality he never makes anybody do anything. He simply gives the performers an opportunity to do what they want to do anyway - be the centre of attention, show off for a bit and get some applause - and then he gives them the script. He tells them exactly what to do to entertain the people, and they are willing to go ahead and do that with enthusiasm. They will enjoy it, too! This is another factor the audience cannot understand because they know that they would not enjoy doing any of those things themselves. So they cannot understand how anybody else could possibly enjoy doing those things either, because they are spectators themselves by nature and have never experienced the buzz a performer gets from being in the spotlight. As a result they might well end up accepting the general suggestion that "the hypnotist made them do it" with the mysterious power of hypnosis. Which isn't even necessary, and also isn't possible. The truth about trance and suggestion is this: whether we're in trance or not – and even if we are in the deepest trance possible - we still only accept suggestions we personally find acceptable.

## But my Boss would never do those things!

Sometimes people reject the statement about suggestions needing to be "acceptable", insisting that: "I *know* him, I work with him every day, he would never behave like that! I'm telling you, that hypnotist had him completely in his power." Once again, you must remember that you may have never seen that person in this particular situation before - not only being given permission but also *encouragement* to behave in a ridiculous fashion, and then rewarded with applause for doing so, thereby being encouraged to continue. The other aspect that most people know nothing about is the attitude of the Subconscious mind towards game-playing scenarios, and its real role in directing our behaviour - which is no mystery to those of us who understand it well and work with it all the time. Throughout this book I have explained in detail what the Subconscious is, how it normally operates and also how hypnotherapists work with it. It becomes clear from all the explanations, examples and case studies that the generalised notion that hypnotists actually control the behaviour of others is laughable. The structure of the stage hypnosis show is designed to convince the audience of something which is not true at all.

The Subconscious mind does not do what it is told, it does what it likes. When participants are on the stage, they know perfectly well they are engaged in a theatrical performance. This is not real life, and they would not behave like this in real life.

That is usually true of all activity in the field of entertainment. To be entertaining, something more than ordinary behaviour is required, obviously. What is required is a performance. In karaoke it is a musical performance, or as near to musical as possible. In stage hypnosis, it is a ridiculous performance. Most people are content to watch a ridiculous performance - they just have no desire to participate in one for the entertainment of others, so they don't join in. But you only have to look at any ordinary holiday 'club rep show' to see that some people do want to do these things, and any kind of formal hypnosis isn't even required, especially if you have alcohol. Given a little alcohol and some encouragement and applause, quite a lot of ordinary people will join in if the circumstances are right. You are on holiday. Hardly anyone here knows you. This is not real life. All bets are off. Sometimes we surprise ourselves. Maybe there is a little bit of a performer in everyone, given the right circumstances.

At various times, our reactions to what is going on around us are either being decided by the conscious mind, or by the Subconscious. Since most people scarcely realize the Subconscious even exists, it is common for the conscious mind to take the attitude that it directs all our behaviour, but it obviously doesn't. Look what happens when you consciously decide you are *not* going to eat chocolate anymore, or you are *not* going to get drunk again, or *not* gamble, *not* see her anymore, *not* eat too much, *not* believe his lies, *not* get another dog. Your actual behaviour goes a different way from the conscious decision because the Subconscious has its own agenda, and it is nowhere near as miserable, sensible and generally killjoy as the conscious mind. Also, the Subconscious does not know about the latest conscious decision or any of the reasons for it, so it does not take any of that into account in directing your behaviour and things continue as before, just as if the decision/promise/resolution had never been made. You can throw willpower at it if you like, but if you have read *The Willpower Myth* already you might prefer not to bother, and just ring a hypnotherapist instead. Why do things the hard way?

All we really do in hypnotherapy is explain to the Subconscious that the habitual gambling behaviour - for example - is now under review, and then explain all the reasons for reconsidering it. These are aspects of the matter the Subconscious has never considered before, even though the conscious mind may have been over and over this ground many times without any change resulting from those analytical exercises. An experienced therapist will go into detail and plead a convincing case for the cessation of gambling behaviour, but without making it sound as if we are laying the law down because that would not work. Even then, the client's Subconscious mind does not *have* to change anything. It does what it chooses to do. It is exactly like arguing a case before a judge - as therapists, we have no power over the judge's decision but if we make it a good case we can win a ruling in favour of the change, and then all compulsive urge to gamble ceases. This always amazes the conscious mind of the former gambler concerned, for two reasons: 1). it didn't expect that to happen, because it never happened before, and 2). because the conscious mind didn't do anything at all, so it cannot understand why anything changed.

The conscious mind is bound by logic and reason, provided we are sane. It has a tendency to be cautious and usually takes into account what other people may think about what we choose to do. By contrast, the Subconscious is creative and imaginative, just as happy with nonsense as with reason, is sometimes impulsive or spontaneous and does not necessarily care at all what other people think. Whenever we make a choice, one or other part of the mind may be 'in the driving seat' as it were, directing our behaviour at the time. Sometimes they can be fighting over the metaphorical steering wheel - this is what is going on when people feel torn: they notice that they are arguing with themselves. The classic cartoon representation is of an angel on one side and a devil on the other. They cannot both win at any one time. When we drink alcohol, the balance quickly tips in favour of the Subconscious. If we drink more, the Subconscious takes over completely and logic, reason and caution can go right out the window.

This does not mean the Subconscious is totally irresponsible, you understand – it certainly is not the devil! It's just that normally its wilder impulsiveness can be tempered by the caution of the conscious mind anyway. Alcohol makes the conscious mind abnormally subdued, giving the Subconscious an unusual amount of clout in the decision-making process. This doesn't make it wicked either, but it can make our behaviour more rash, as anyone who likes a drink will be well aware. We can get a bit more carried away than we usually would. And if anyone has anger or violence in them – or criminal tendencies - those can be unleashed as well. Alcohol doesn't cause the anger, or the criminal tendencies. Something else did that. Alcohol just makes it more difficult to inhibit.

People drink alcohol to go into trance, they just don't realize that. There are many routes into trance - alcohol is just one of the various chemical ones. The intoxicated state of trance is different from natural trance, too. Boozy trance can be maudlin, clumsy or belligerent, whereas natural trance is generally positive and a pleasant frame of mind. Yet natural trance can bear some other temporary similarities to inebriation, so the people taking part in the stage hypnosis performance will tend to be more impulsive once they are in trance. They will be quite happy with nonsense and silliness, more imaginative and pretty unlikely to ponder, whilst they are still in trance, what anyone in the audience thinks about what they are doing. If the hypnotist has selected the right kind of candidates then they are unlikely to care about that later either. The ones who are usually shy will probably be quite high on the fact that their shyness seemed to vanish whilst they were exploring their new role as an entertainer. And the ones who are not shy - the outgoing livewires - don't much care what happens as long as everyone is laughing and clapping. They certainly won't waste any time later worrying about what anyone else thinks of their antics. And why should they?

Once these people are up on the stage, they know they are there to entertain the people and they have accepted that role. They also know the drill because they have seen it all before on TV, which is why they don't really need 'prepping'. They already expect that if the stage hypnotist turns to them, under those circumstances, snaps his fingers and commands them to "Sleep!" the correct response is to close the eyes and slump as if suddenly dormant. They certainly do not have to react like that but any other response would be inappropriate if they are to avoid being a spoilsport and they have already chosen to play a sporting role in the hypnotist's show. If they do not respond, or they choose to do something else, they have broken that entertainment contract and then they cannot be an entertainer. Instead they will be dismissed from the stage right away and thus demoted to mere spectator again. The audience will not be impressed by their non-compliance, the hypnotist will not be pleased – in short, *no-one will like them if they bugger up the show,* unless the crowd don't like the hypnotist. So just by virtue of being in that position they have every motivation to respond appropriately and therefore no self-interest in hesitating or resisting the suggestion.

Now, the above explanation makes it seem as if I am talking about a conscious choice here, as if they are thinking all this through. No, the conscious mind is already a bystander once they are the centre of attention. The real world has disappeared, now we are in Magic Land, but the conscious mind is still rather too close to the driving seat for the stage hypnotist to be sure it is not going to interfere at some stage, so he will be inclined soon to give the conscious mind some proper down-time, so that the Subconscious mind will feel free to really have fun, and not be bothered by conscious doubts or niggles. Just like when you've had a few vodkas, in fact.

The quickest way to do this is with a shock induction. Shock inductions are instant, and really just take advantage of a defensive mechanism in our mental control systems. As I have mentioned elsewhere, if something unexpected happens the Subconscious may instantly assume full control, and this is what happens instantly if something 'makes us jump'. A shock induction doesn't need to be deeply shocking, although the same thing would certainly happen if it was. The fact is that any sudden movement or contact that momentarily takes someone by surprise will cause their Subconscious to sit up and take notice, especially if developments seem unpredictable or unfamiliar, or if several things are happening at once so there is some degree of confusion, which is often the case if you are the centre of attention in a live and unscripted show. All the hypnotist needs to do is clap you smartly on the shoulder or snap his fingers fairly close to you and your Subconscious mind will assume full control. The conscious mind is completely relieved of command and has little influence over your behaviour from that point onwards. Sometime later when the Subconscious decides to delegate behavioural control once again to the conscious mind – when you 'snap out of it' it then returns to its default position of paying far less attention to the outside world.

It is standard practice with a shock induction to present the Subconscious with a simple suggestion it instantly recognises just a split second after it takes full control, otherwise the opportunity to give the conscious mind 'free drinks at the bar' for the rest of the performance, as it were, might pass too soon. What word is instantaneously recognisable in every hypnosis show you ever saw? "Sleep!" The Subconscious knows exactly how to respond to that: it is being directed to switch off conscious awareness, leaving only Subconscious awareness. Bear in mind that the Subconscious mind of a human being will have no issue with doing that under ordinary circumstances – it does it regularly. It can always switch it back on again if need be, it doesn't need an instruction. So if that suggestion is abruptly fired at the Subconscious at that precise moment, it may well be happy to comply provided there is no apparent disadvantage in doing so.

Let me be very clear about one thing. That will happen only if it seems appropriate and everything is as it should be. The Subconscious will not respond to that if it is not happy about something. The person will only respond to that if they really don't have any objection to playing a role in the show, i.e. they are prepared to trust the hypnotist and these proceedings are pretty much what they would expect in these circumstances. They do not have to go deeper into trance, and they don't have to stay there either. It is optional. But since trance is a stress-free mental state in which deep states of relaxation are easily accessed, it does have obvious appeal. Once you experience that for yourself, you aren't in any hurry to leave that deep state because it is a pleasant feeling. And if you are obliged to leave it at some stage and become more active for a while, you are always more than happy to return to it, which is why it is so easy for the hypnotist to elicit that response anytime after that by repeating the signal "sleep". The shock element is no longer required by then.

It seems that people differ quite a bit in terms of just how much conscious processing (analytical thinking) ceases following these suggestions. Obviously all of them are aware subconsciously of what happens after that, so in that sense they are never unaware. Some people retain conscious awareness completely: they just feel relaxed and a bit detached from ordinary reality, which is a pleasant state of conscious dissociation. This is still a trance but it is a fairly light state and sometimes these people feel like they are not really in a trance, they are just going along with the activities because it seems harmless enough. Some participants realise that they know what is happening perfectly well but aren't sure why they are doing the things that they are doing, and may feel a bit bemused by it all. They may also drift out of trance at some stage, possibly even opting out of the performance before the end of the show. But most of them will stick with it because they feel obliged to do so and don't really mind anyway. At the other end of the scale there are people who go very deep, reaching the level of trance known as somnambulism, which literally means 'sleepwalking'.

Clearly there are similarities between hypnotic somnambulism and actual sleep-walking: they may even be the same state. The Subconscious never sleeps, but in both these states the conscious mind is not engaging with external reality, so it is effectively a dreaming state yet the body is mobile, unlike in ordinary sleep when bodily movement is minimal or discontinued. None of these changes are ever truly under the control of the hypnotist even though he behaves as if they are, but always under the direct control of the other person's Subconscious mind. It is also the Subconscious that decides when to re-activate conscious activity.

## The Dimmer Switch

I tend to think of the Subconscious mind's control of conscious activity as a bit like a dimmer switch for an electric light, it can be moved to any level or switched off completely, and not everybody's 'switches' will be operated in the same way when presented with suggestions by another person. Certainly the conscious mind does not control it, and when we are treating insomnia with hypnotherapy we are essentially just asking the Subconscious to be more consistent about the pattern of switching conscious awareness on and off completely. (There's more to it than that, but that's another issue.)

Even in ordinary sleep there are times when the conscious mind is re-activated briefly, or partially engaged so that we might be dimly aware of something on a conscious level too. When someone is soundly asleep it seems that the conscious mind is more or less switched off, whereas in trance states like somnambulism it is in such a relaxed state that this creates a very similar effect: the conscious mind is doing virtually nothing. Although we commonly assure clients that hypnosis is not sleep, this is mainly in order to remove conscious expectations caused by stage hypnosis. This is important because the vast majority of clients will not feel as if they are asleep when they are in trance, especially if they are nervous because they are new to hypnotherapy. Some may not allow themselves to relax much at first, but this quickly changes as they become familiar with the process and realise it is all very easy.

## In therapy, we do NOT want the conscious mind switched OFF!

In the very deep hypnotic states - in which conscious analytical activity would just seem like way too much effort - there may be very little difference between sleep states and deep trance. What is interesting is that if the client does actually fall asleep for real – which rarely happens - **suggestions presented to them after that are not acted upon**, including directions to emerge from trance. This is because they are no longer in trance, they are asleep. It then becomes necessary to waken them as you would any person sleeping soundly, with a gentle shake of the shoulder, a klaxon or a bucket of cold water.

This raises an interesting question: as the Subconscious remains active during sleep states anyway, why doesn't the Subconscious mind of a sleeping client respond to suggestions presented in the usual way, just like the client in trance? At first this led me to wonder if some aspect of the conscious mind is involved in the change process, so if it is shut down completely, perhaps an active link to the Subconscious becomes inactive. But now I suspect it is because there is an oversimplification in the notion of a conscious mind and a Subconscious mind. It is all one mind really - and clearly there is different mental activity going on in all these different states.

In hypnotherapy, for purely practical reasons we have a 'model' of the human mind which divides up control responsibilities according to what each side of the mind can evidently fix. If a person cannot solve their own problem through conscious efforts, this is apparently not under conscious control. This becomes a safer assumption when we observe that other clients also report the same limitation. If we then ask the Subconscious to fix it and it does – and especially if we try this with numerous clients and get consistent success that way - it becomes a pretty safe assumption that the Subconscious mind controls that, which is precisely why the conscious efforts were in vain.

## "I've tried and tried, but I can't do it!"

How many people assume that their previous conscious efforts to solve their problem are 'failure', or concluded that solving the problem must be a terribly difficult thing to do? Having no practical knowledge of the Subconscious mind, all too often they will then miserably accept that they *cannot change that,* when what they should really be concluding is that *they cannot change that merely through conscious efforts.* This is a much more scientific conclusion because it is more precise. A successful appeal to the Subconscious mind proves – as we find time and time again – that *it* can change it quite easily, it had just never been asked to do so and was quite unaware of any conscious resolutions or efforts to change it before.

## The Simple Usefulness of Trance States

In non-trance states the Subconscious mind tends not to bother with the world around us, as the conscious mind is already attending to it. That would change instantly if we received a shock or an injury, but otherwise there is no need for the Subconscious to involve itself in everyday social stuff, that's the conscious mind's domain. This effectively means that if we want to present a request for change to the Subconscious mind, trance is a pre-requisite or it will not even be aware of the request!

So trance states facilitate the presentation of the case for change but the normal state of sleep seems to slow down the absorption of information considerably. It doesn't quite shut it down: it has been previously demonstrated that tape-recorded information can be learned by the Subconscious during sleep if it is replayed on many occasions. However, it takes a long time to do this, and hypnotherapy doesn't normally take a long time. I suspect that the problem with the sleep state – for hypnotherapists - is not so much that the conscious mind is not active in sleep but that some key part of the Subconscious also disengages in that state, but not in trance.

I like to make it clear when I am speculating and I am certainly doing that here. I have often stated that the Subconscious "is not analytical". Sometimes I qualify that by stating that "the Subconscious is not analytical in the way the conscious mind is", which I think is more accurate. Hypnotherapists know from experience that the client's Subconscious mind will *consider* a request for change. How do we know? Because the range of possible responses includes: immediate positive response (the usual outcome), partial response, hesitant response, response followed by back-tracking, an initial delay and then a response, no response at all and an emphatic rejection (the symptoms become more pronounced). Further requests for change can easily improve matters if necessary. All this capability indicates that the Subconscious mind has opinions, doesn't obey orders and can be persuaded to change its view in precisely the same way as the conscious mind can: through the presentation of a sound case for change.

## The Stage Show and Memory

One of the things the conscious mind normally does (when it is active) is to create a temporary, rough recording of recent events. This is what we call "short-term memory". In sound sleep, in deep states of trance and also in the latter stages of drunkenness the conscious mind stops bothering to do this, which explains why some people have no conscious memory of certain parts of their stage hypnosis performance, their hypnotherapy session or their taxi journey home after the office party. When alcohol is involved this is sometimes called a "blackout" - an unnecessarily dramatic term for what is actually an ordinary enough phenomenon, which amounts to nothing more than extreme laziness on the part of the conscious mind. If it happens a lot though, you are probably drinking excessively which a good hypnotherapist can fix for you quite easily as long as they have plenty of experience dealing with that issue. Sometimes this involves clearing emotional issues too, if there is a link. That might take a few sessions but it is better than liver failure.

## The Fear of Not Remembering

Some people in the audience might find the idea of not remembering part of the stage hypnosis proceedings scary - but then they would probably find the idea of being on the stage scary anyway, so they wouldn't choose to join in. Most people who opt to join in with all this are lively sorts who just enjoy being at the centre of the action. They don't analyse any of this but they are already Subconsciously aware that if they don't respond in a suitable manner, then they obviously aren't going to be in the limelight for very long. Since their main motivation is to show off and get some attention and applause, they are very likely to go ahead and do what they know is required of them. They do have a choice. They could resist all suggestion and say: "Har har, you can't hypnotise me!" But where would that get them? The audience would not be impressed because that is the behaviour of a spoilsport, and their status would immediately diminish from:

> *Comedy player, centre of attention and potential star of the show!*

> to: spoilsport and nobody.

Why would they want to do that? Don't forget, these lively types are *excited* to be playing a part in the show. They are aware of the audience's expectations and they crave the approval of the audience, signalled through laughter and applause. They are not going to do anything to spoil the show. All the cynics and spoilsports who *would* want to ruin the show have been left in their seats, or have already been returned to their seats by the stage hypnotist. The ones that remain are right onside with the hypnotist in wanting it to be a good show and aiming to play a key part in it.

## The Normally Shy Type

Those players who are usually shy in social situations actually find relief from that shyness in the unreality of the stage setting and also in the state of trance. The deeper in trance they go the more comfortable they feel. Relaxation clearly enhances the welcome change, so that these individuals feel very different in a hypnosis performance to the way they ordinarily feel in social situations. They feel free to act quite spontaneously, whereas their usual social demeanour is anxious and hesitant. This is caused by the conscious mind's fretful inhibitions, which disappear once the Subconscious mind is in the driving seat! This can be such a new-found freedom for them that it feels quite intoxicating, even euphoric. They'll play any daft game you like as long as it means they can go on feeling like this. Of course it still has to all make sense within the context of a stage hypnosis show – it all has to be silly fun and games with no serious implications in the real world. If the stage hypnotist started suggesting things that were out of context, then the Subconscious would cease to respond and might well decide to turn up the level of analytical processing so the conscious mind could figure out why things had apparently changed – in other words, the player would emerge from trance without instruction to do so. The Subconscious isn't stupid, and has safety and security as its top priorities.

## The Team is Now Assembled

So by going through a subtle selection process the stage hypnotist has stacked the deck in his favour because all the people who would probably refuse or hesitate to respond to the fun suggestions he will later put forward have been eliminated from the set. He is left with exactly the right people for this sort of performance. If he has done that with slick stage professionalism and confidence, the audience will be unlikely to have noticed that these people have been carefully selected in reality. Everyone else has either excluded themselves or been weeded out without explanation, or with a cursory and misleading suggestion such as "I can't work with you", which accounts for the false notion that some people "can't be hypnotised".

Ideally the audience should have accepted the notion that this is a fairly random selection and be generally unaware that these people are different from them - not in terms of being more 'susceptible', more easily influenced or 'hypnotizable' - but in terms of their personal feelings about the opportunity to be a performer in this show here tonight. They may not be professional performers but they are performers at heart, or prepared to give it a go – which actually quite a lot of people are if given the right opportunity, as evidenced by the popularity of karaoke. This factor entirely explains their willingness to perform all kinds of craziness by the end of the show which non-performers regard as bizarre because they would have a strong aversion to doing that sort of thing themselves.

No *desire* to perform means that such a person is a non-performer, whether hypnotised or not. The hypnotist does not want any of those people on the stage, because although he might find it easy enough to hypnotise some of them, they would not respond to the crazy suggestions. Or produce a very lukewarm response which amounts to a poor show. No, he wants those people to remain in the audience where they belong - but he doesn't want them to understand that aspect of the selection process. To complete the illusion he needs the individual audience members to *imagine* all the way through the show: "If he could get me up there, maybe he could make me behave like that with the mysterious power of hypnosis! Look, he is controlling those people's minds: they are doing exactly what he is telling them to do!"

Actually they are not doing those things because the hypnotist says so or even because they are in hypnosis, but because *they enjoy doing things like that* - even if they have never really had a chance to discover that before this opportunity came up. And although some of the suggestions are spoken as if they are commands – such as "Sleep!" - they remain mere suggestions. That person could open their eyes and walk off the stage anytime they like - but they probably won't because they are right where they want to be already. In truth they are just having fun.

Now, that is the factor the majority of the audience are unlikely to appreciate because they would not enjoy doing any of those things themselves, so they cannot imagine how anyone else could. But that is just the difference between performers and spectators... no more mysterious than the fact that a few people love to be the centre of attention where there is a big crowd, but most people dread it. Also, the audience might be under the impression that the performers are making fools of themselves because they are imagining themselves in the same situation and cringing. But that is not what the performers think, they think they are entertaining everyone and all the laughter and applause is for them so it encourages them. Some of them at least will be getting a real buzz out of this, especially if they know the show is going to be on television.

Have you ever been in a situation where you know millions of people are going to be watching you and hearing what you say? If you are horrified by the thought, you are not a performer at heart. You may have talents, but the desire to perform is a quite separate thing. If you are thrilled at the thought of having an audience of millions, then you have the soul of a performer even if you haven't an ounce of talent. If you have talent as well, then you have real potential in the world of entertainment and/or politics. In fact quite a lot of natural born performers skip the talent bit and still do quite well in those fields. Sheer brass neck and front count for a lot in public affairs, especially now that sense has been largely replaced by images and soundbites.

Simply being one of life's performers, though, does not necessarily mean that you would choose to take part in a stage hypnotism performance. It is still a matter of personal taste and stage hypnotism is not to everyone's taste. It depends upon illusion to present itself as 'mind control by somebody else' but this false impression also accounts for some of the disapproval or discomfort in the minds of some audience members. Thoughts of "Look at what the hypnotist has made that poor young man do!" coupled with the notion that the young man seems only semi-aware of his situation can offend spectators of a milder nature because they feel for the poor guy... completely unaware that he is probably having a good time. They are projecting their personal discomfort onto him, but it is an empathy for which he has no use, and of which he would also be completely unaware! If he got up there of his own accord, he volunteered himself as a player because he wanted to play and that is why he is engaging in that imaginative activity. If someone watching the performance is uncomfortable, that discomfort isn't really compassion. It starts and ends with that spectator, which is exactly why they are not joining in themselves. It is quite possible to enjoy watching though, and as long as the show is just ridiculous and not cruel, we can safely assume the performers are enjoying themselves, or at least don't mind.

People who prefer the spectator's role may never know what it feels like to win huge rounds of applause from hundreds of people, star in a TV show or be bathed in mass approval like "that poor young man" on the stage. Still they are free to enjoy the entertainment, thus fulfilling their true role as a spectator.

## In Summary

So really there are two things going on in stage hypnosis shows. There is what is really happening upon the stage, which is just an elaborate game for players in which their Subconscious minds may well respond to ideas put forward by the top banana - the main player, the hypnotist. Or it may not, but it probably will because they wouldn't have bothered getting up there in the first place if they had no intention of playing the game.

Then there is what the audience *thinks* is going on up there - which is actually only going on in their own imagination, led by the suggestions of the hypnotist. They do not realise this because they think they are watching the hypnotist fool *other people,* they do not realise they are being deeply misled themselves with words like 'sleep'. Sleep is a different state. Trance is a waking state, and we know that sleeping people do not respond to the presentation of information unless it is repeated day after day over weeks, such as a tape recording being replayed many times. On the stage, the word 'sleep' is being used deliberately to create a false impression in the minds of the audience. Whether the guy on the stage reckons he is hypnotised or not is neither here nor there: the only thing that really matters is how he feels about being on the stage and playing the role of an entertainer for a little while.

Remember that some of the suggestions are aimed at the audience, but they don't realise that. Words like 'sleep' and 'under' are clever, misleading directions to the audience to create a false impression, to suggest a mystery where there isn't one really. The hypnotist is trying to convince the audience that these players are in some sort of mysterious state of mind the audience have never been in, which is untrue. Trance is a normal state of mind we drift in and out of all the time. Whatever we call it – daydreaming, reverie, hypnosis, mesmerism, fascination, being riveted or enthralled – it is always the same state and familiar to us all. The expression "under hypnosis" doesn't mean a thing in reality, but it cleverly suggests: 'under' a spell, 'under' my power. These connections are made Subconsciously in the minds of the audience, and many of them will also make an instant connection with 'under' anaesthetic, assuming that "those people are completely 'under', they don't know what is going on!"

Of course they know what is going on. What they are paying attention to may vary quite a bit and the conscious mind may wander off sometimes but there is nothing peculiar about that, it happens often. Levels of trance and relaxation may vary a lot between players, and the resultant conscious laziness may affect the degree of conscious recall later in some people – just like drunkenness can – but the players know what they are doing at the time and don't have to do any of it, just as they didn't have to participate in the first place. It is all voluntary and even though our behaviour when in trance is being directed by the Subconscious, that does not make us 'more suggestible' as I have already explained: it simply means that our primary interests have switched to the Subconscious agenda for the time being. The suggestions still have to have some appeal - or else the performance generally has to have appeal - or that person would not do those things no matter how deep in trance they were.

For the small percentage who go really deep whilst on stage, the experience will be a bit like sleepwalking or talking in your sleep – a dreamier experience - and the hypnotist needs to handle those people diligently. They are not asleep but they are close to it because their conscious mind is hardly doing anything, so their dissociation from reality is greater. They could snap out of it any time they like, but they probably won't because it is very relaxing and enjoyable to go that deep into trance states. However, their Subconscious mind is in charge of that decision, not the hypnotist.

Even though the hypnotist is putting on a performance of being in control of other people, don't forget he is a performer too and playing a central role in the creation of the illusion that he is controlling others. Most people in stage shows never go particularly deep anyway and are really just larking about and having a good time being the centre of attention. They are likely to be in some kind of trance even if it is not a deep one, but that is not why they are putting on a performance. They are doing that mainly for attention and applause.

So the stage hypnotist is not controlling anybody. In reality he is simply orchestrating an imaginary game and passing it off as something entirely different. The stage hypnotist would certainly prefer to be the only person present who knows about trance states, the Subconscious agenda and how to get latent entertainers to perform. They usually don't need much encouragement.

## Case Mysteries No.9: Problems with Groups and Couples

As I've mentioned elsewhere in the book, people often assume that for hypnotherapy to work, you've got to really want it to work. This is not entirely wrong in the sense that if you actually *don't* want it to work, change is rather less likely - but then that would not be failure anyway, since the person got what they wanted. No change.

The question really reflects our general assumption that you will have to try hard to get success in anything, you need motivation and effort. Certainly if you are completely unmotivated - like the type I refer to as The Totally Emotionless - positive response is quite unlikely but those people are pretty unusual. The truth is that in hypnotherapy you do not need much motivation at all to get a perfectly good response. In fact as long as the Subconscious has no objection to the change and the therapist can make a reasonable case to the Subconscious for an advantage in making that change, very often that will do fine.

This point about motivation has become a bone of contention recently for hypnotherapists when it comes to advertising, because Advertising Standards people have gradually placed more and more restrictions upon what we are allowed to tell people we can do with hypnotherapy. Instead of "Smoking Cessation" we now have to use an expression such as: "Help With Stopping Smoking", or where we might have once preferred "Stop Smoking in One Session!" we now have to say things like: "If you *really* want to stop smoking, then one session could be all you need!"

These restrictions are supposedly to protect the public but actually they are misleading because it gives the public the impression that willpower is still needed even with hypnotherapy - which is not true. However, the advertising standards people do not know that. And of course they are being leaned on by medical authorities, who are generally both ignorant about and prejudiced against hypnotherapy.

They don't want people to get their hopes up, you see. They seem to imagine that ordinary people are terribly delicate and might go all to pieces if something they try doesn't really come off, or doesn't happen straight away. In my experience the majority of people are not like that at all, but really rather robust and practical, not easily discouraged and quite able to be positive and persistent enough to achieve success, especially with the right help and encouragement.

Sometimes though, other forces are in play and this is particularly so when people come for therapy in twos and threes. Couples, friends, work colleagues, that sort of thing. Over the years, I have conducted hypnotherapy sessions on a one-to-one basis, worked with people in pairs, in small groups, and in larger groups, and I have to say there is no doubt in my mind that the highest success rate for smoking is the one-to-one session, where the client simply decided to get rid of the habit independently of external pressures, and didn't feel the need to rope some other smoker they know into the procedure as well.

This is because the involvement of other persons can complicate matters on an emotional level. It is understandable that people who know nothing about hypnotherapy might assume that they may benefit from some 'moral support', or that it will be easier to stay free afterwards if their husband or best friend quits at the same time. But they are looking at hypnotherapy as if it were the same as all the other quitting methods: as if there is an endurance element to it after the session, during which troubled times it would be helpful to have a fellow sufferer to go through the process with, like having a buddy to work out with down at the gym.

I can tell that many people are expecting these difficulties to be there after the session because of the way they talk about the success story that inspired them to book a session with me in the first place:

"Yes, Frank and I wanted to come and see you because Patricia - our next door neighbour - came to you six months ago and she's still doing really well... and I'm amazed, because she was an even heavier smoker than me, and I never thought *she* would stop!"

Ok, several things wrong with that. First of all, I think I'll let Frank speak for himself in due course, with regard to how much *he* really wanted to come and see me, or even wants to quit. If a couple are quitting together, the decision and the motivation behind it are never evenly balanced, there is always a prime mover. And by asking them - individually and privately - who decided on this particular quitting attempt and who decided upon the hypnotherapy approach, it is usually the prime mover who will insist that "We *both* decided!" whereas the smoker with the rope-marks around their neck may answer with rather less certainty.

Ironically – and this will surprise you, I'm sure – if one of them has difficulties after the first session it is more often the prime mover that has the problem rather than the one who probably wouldn't have come at all, left to themselves. Difficulties are not failure, by the way, so the complication can usually be sorted out later. But it is interesting that the person with apparently *more motivation* is also more likely to have the conflict that temporarily delays their success. It is precisely because they are more worked up about the issue that their emotional response in the first session can be conflicted, causing a hesitation that requires correction afterwards. Not caring much either way can actually be a bit of a plus in hypnotherapy, though you wouldn't expect it.

Secondly, Patricia is *not* "still doing really well", she is a non-smoker. She has simply been returned to normal: tobacco is useless and meaningless to her once again, just as it was in the first place. Anything less than that is not total success and no decent hypnotherapist would be satisfied by anything less than absolute success where smoking is concerned because there is a risk of backsliding later on if matters are left like that. I always tell my new non-smokers, at the end of the session:

"What we expect now is total success. That means no desire to smoke, no need for willpower in any situation, perfectly comfortable around other people whether they smoke or not, no cravings whatsoever, no bad moods, no over-eating and no weight gain, in fact absolutely delighted with the results and happy for all changes to be permanent. As long as we have all that, I'm happy, we're done." Then I add, with emphasis: "If you have any difficulty whatsoever, at any time, I expect you to ring me because I would know exactly what to do about it should that occur."

So I ask the newcomer, did Patricia explain the difference hypnotherapy made, in her experience? And sure enough: "Oh, she is amazed, from the moment she left your office she has never wanted one, and she sits with us in the pub, and she says it never bothers her. And obviously it doesn't, I mean I've seen Pat try to quit numerous times and it always used to drive her up the wall, but not this time. Everybody is amazed! Yes, she has done really well."

Correct! She *has done* really well. She responded perfectly to the session and from the moment she left the office she has not had to make any effort to maintain that. The previous statement "She *is doing* really well" assumes an ongoing effort that simply does not exist when we have the proper response to the first session. This is quite different from any other quitting method. Willpower is genuinely not required in hypnotherapy, and since willpower is a conscious effort anyway it is quite outside the area in which hypnotherapy effectively operates.

So if a person rings me after a smoking session to say they still have a problem, then *we ain't done yet,* it is as simple as that. And the chances of that happening are significantly higher if their first session was not wholly and exclusively about that individual, which is why working with couples or groups is more problematic than one-to-one sessions.

One final thing needs mentioning, concerning the new client's assumptions about Patricia: "I'm amazed, because she was an even heavier smoker than me..." This suggests that success with hypnotherapy is more surprising if someone smoked heavily than if they did not smoke much. This is actually a common assumption but to those of us who understand compulsive habits it is laughable, and really comes back to the old notion of addiction, as if the heavy smoker 'needs' all that smoke, just because the initial impulse to reach for tobacco *feels* like a need. Actually it is just an impulse: a prompt from the Subconscious mind. Once it is shut down, there is no impulse to do it at all.

Nobody needs anything in the smoke - never did, and never will. Not eighty times a day, not sixty, not twenty, not once. No more than anyone genuinely needs to wash their hands forty times a day, lose twenty quid on a bad racing tip or eat a giant Toblerone. They might feel *compelled* to do any one of those things... but since hypnotherapy can remove the compulsions, they do not even need to put up with that, let alone fight a battle with themselves over it. Nothing wrong with Toblerones by the way, I'm not suggesting they are a problem. It is the compulsive urges we can do without. Of course you want the freedom to eat a Toblerone, you just don't want to feel compelled to do it. Although they are a bit weird, aren't they? Toblerones, I mean. They taste quite nice but you can't eat them without hurting yourself. Pointy, angular chocolate – whose guilt-ridden idea was that?

## When People Want to Quit Together

Now, I could relate any number of interesting cases about couples and colleagues, groups and various joint efforts to quit smoking or lose weight. Nowadays I never do group therapy, nor do I work with more than one person at a time but I still have the problem of colleagues or couples wanting to quit on the same day, usually booking their sessions back to back. I do advise them that having sessions on different days is preferable but most do not like the idea because they have it fixed in their head that quitting should be synchronized, if only because of the assumption that they will be 'tempted' to smoke if the other person is still smoking, even if it is only for a couple of days. I suppose nearly everybody assumes this whether they are a smoker or not, because they do not realise hypnotherapy eliminates any 'urge' to smoke, so they will not feel tempted at all once the whole process has truly been completed to my satisfaction. But I don't put any smoker under pressure to do things my way. Having explained the facts, I will organise sessions according to the clients' preference, even if it is not my preference.

You may be wondering at this point *why* immediate success might be less certain if they both attend on the same occasion. Well, first of all let me explain why group therapy is not the best approach to smoking cessation, because these things are linked. The fact is people behave differently when in groups from the way they would behave in a one-to-one encounter. This is partly because they are more self-conscious when others are there, and so some of their responses are actually adjusted to take account of the presence of others, and what *their* opinions might be. Also, some people feel intimidated by others, especially if some of them are outspoken, and may withdraw emotionally and feel 'left out' or inferior (both negative states of mind). Unfortunately the therapist cannot do enough to reverse this whilst others are making stronger demands for attention.

## Negative Associations

Group situations organised around an instructor or 'teaching' figure immediately recall school for many people, and if that was not a time of easy success and advancement for them, this creates a tension and uncertainty which makes some people defensive and that is completely the wrong mood for effective hypnotherapy. Also, childhood is a time of vulnerability and trepidation, during which there is a lack of power and very little personal choice, thus inevitably some resentment towards 'parental' and guiding figures generally. Consequently there can be a tendency to rebel in some individuals, as they regress emotionally into youthful attitudes. This may manifest in a tendency not to take the guiding figure very seriously, disagree or just mess about, cracking jokes and wasting time. Yes, many adults slide into this very easily as soon as you put them in a group and try to teach them something - just ask the poor sod running the local *Weightwatchers* class, they'll know exactly what I'm talking about. But hardly any adults will do that in a one to one situation. The atmosphere is completely different.

In addition, people's opinions, feelings and experiences differ and it is too easy for a debate to get going within the group about varying personal views that really do not matter at the end of the day but that sort of petty disagreement can cause friction, negativity and discord within the group. It certainly wastes time, and the more time is wasted the less therapy is being provided.

Then there is the element of competition. Those that seem keen to learn and eager to respond can irritate the ones who are not feeling so positive, causing them to take up an even more negative position, so that their input can then become a negative influence on the more average members of the group, as well as making them less likely to succeed themselves. In fact there are so many ways that the group dynamics can work against success where smoking is concerned that you might as well forget it. There is no advantage for hypnotherapists in taking on more than one smoker at a time *except* the financial advantage, but since the success rate is significantly compromised by group dynamics, even that is questionable.

Any suggestion that people might help to motivate one another positively by tackling the problem together is even more laughable with smokers than it is with dieters – smokers are probably more likely to encourage one another to relapse at some stage than to succeed, partly because of the way we all started smoking in the first place – *in groups,* doing something that we shouldn't and laughing at the people who advised against it.

Some of this happens with people in twos and threes as well, so it is easy for the whole thing to come off the rails in a way that is easily avoided simply by dealing with people one at a time. Where couples are concerned, dealing with them together can be really difficult because the petty disagreements and differences of many years can find their way into the discussion, and again there is the element of competition. Smokers usually do not expect hypnotherapy to be successful anyway, and if a couple are doing it together there is an added pressure. These are typical of the Subconscious fears:

> "What if he is successful and I'm not?" Or:

> "What if I stop smoking, and he *doesn't* - that would be typical of him, when he suggested this in the first place! I can see it now, I'll have stopped and he'll still be puffing away..."

These are just a few of the conflicts that are distracting people and causing uncertainty when another smoker is involved. If both smokers attend the same session, the very presence of the other person can be a distraction during the trance section because people find themselves wondering what the other person thinks of what the therapist is saying instead of simply responding to it themselves.

N.B.: I know I have stated elsewhere that it doesn't matter what a person *thinks consciously* during a session but these distractions can cause emotional conflicts and create a mood of uncertainty and hesitancy, and that can certainly stall our Subconscious response to positive suggestion. Then again, some people don't respond immediately themselves because they are *waiting to see* if the other person responded. It is a distraction that takes their mind off in a useless circular direction of hesitancy and uncertainty.

So if friends or couples do decide to come along on the same day, even though these days I would no longer attempt to work with them both in the same session, some of these conflicts and distractions are still going to be there. So it can mean that one or both of them may need a second session later to achieve complete success, just because they decided that they had to take this step together regardless of my initial advice. On the other hand, one of them might never have bothered to take the step at all if they hadn't been roped in by the keen one, so it's all swings and roundabouts. And all that matters in the end, I suppose, is that tobacco is ditched successfully by both of them, even if it did take a bit longer because there was more than one Subconscious mind involved.

Occasionally though, roping someone else in just does not work, and I would like to illustrate this with the very memorable case of:

## The Bosses

Some people come to the conclusion, at some point in their lives, that working for other people 'sucks'... as the Americans rather unpleasantly put it. So they decide to set up their own business, be their own boss and make themselves rich. Duncan and Jacquie were two such intrepid folk, and by the time Jacquie telephoned me to arrange Stop Smoking sessions for each of them, they had been pretty successful in doing exactly that. They wouldn't describe themselves as "rich", because nobody does. The richer you get, the more time you spend with even richer people who make your own empire seem puny, until you get to the point where you know people who own islands and it all gets completely mad. Still, they were doing very nicely in their business and were "not short of a bob or two", as people still say in my part of the world even though there has been no such thing as a 'bob' (UK shilling) for many decades.

The Bosses had a couple of factories that made stuff, and they were very busy. By this stage in their empire-building they employed lots of other people to do the actual manufacturing, so they didn't make anything themselves anymore except money. Instead, they managed and directed and planned and had meetings and saw clients and won contracts and negotiated and tendered and moved forward with new products and new markets and forecasts and finance and all the time both smoking 60 a day. The financial cost of smoking wasn't a problem, of course - they had plenty of money. It was just that having come this far, it would be a bit of a shame to drop dead one day right in the middle of an important meeting, and all those ciggies were making that look quite likely, actually.

So Jacquie took the initiative and organised two sessions, setting aside four hours of their valuable time for the purpose of avoiding an inconvenient smoking-related early death. She came in first, leaving Duncan to run the ship single-handed for a couple of hours. Then she would rush back to take over the helm whilst he 'swung by' later. (I love these Americanisms, don't you?)

Jacquie was great. She was bright, she was bold, she was confident. And she was interested - aiming and intending to be successful – but she was tough. No messing with this lady, she interrupted from time to time without hesitation and with no apology, firing questions when she didn't quite get something, and she needed convincing that the details were correct. She was not going to accept anything just because I said so. But she was also quick on the uptake, so that was fine. She had completely the wrong idea about hypnotherapy of course, but that is almost universal, so no surprises there. Yet she adapted easily to the reality, and I could see why she was dynamic and successful. This lady was sharp.

Jacquie honestly believed, when she walked in, that she was a nicotine addict and also that smoking helped her cope with the considerable demands of her normal working day. But before the trance part of the session began she had totally changed that view, and was delighted and astonished by my detailed explanations of why that was not true. The trance section went smoothly too, and Jacquie left my office - I have no doubt - a non-smoker.

Whether she remained a non-smoker is another question, because Jacquie had been quite insistent that she could only do this if Duncan did it too, and if she chose to cling to that idea later it may have caused trouble, because Duncan was a non-starter. Very often though, when I am working with couples, I do my best to get them to dissociate their own quitting-procedure from any thoughts of their partner's outcome. This is how I usually put it across:

> "You know, it's understandable that people want to make this change together... when couples are sharing so many things... sharing their home, their time, sharing their resources, along life's journey... but I need you now to *separate*, in your mind, your own smoking habit and what we are doing here today, from your husband's habit. Because they are actually two separate matters... and his experiences and feelings about all this may be quite different from your own. I need you to focus entirely on your own experience now, because although you two share many things in life, the fact is (and here I will look them directly in the eye) if you get lung cancer you're going through that on your own. You can't share that."

That usually serves to focus the mind, especially for anyone over thirty-five. Jacquie acknowledged the point without hesitation, just as she readily accepted every point that made perfect sense once she understood it clearly.

Duncan was a different kettle of fish altogether. He entered the room in a rush, as if this appointment was probably the least important thing he had to do today, and his manner was brusque. I asked how he was today, and this was how he answered:

"Oh... alright. Just had to tear someone off a strip! Some clown not doing his job properly – nothing unusual there! Almost every day I have to tear someone off a strip. But that's how to get things done, I don't suffer fools gladly. If someone needs telling, they get told - I don't care if it upsets 'em. I don't pay people to make a mess of things."

All this was delivered as if it was some sort of a warning. He sprawled back in the armchair regarding me suspiciously, his thumb propping up his chin and with his fingers splayed across his mouth and nose, a very guarded and surly pose.

## The Importance of Rapport in Hypnotherapy

I believe it was Liebault who first pointed out the significance of rapport: the trust relationship between the 'hypnotizer' and the 'hypnotized'. The dictionary definition of *rapport* is "harmony and agreement". In hypnotherapy practice, establishing rapport comes down to finding a way to get on with the client and avoid conflict, and it is very important to establish effective rapport as early as possible in the session so that the communication process goes well.

So I tried. Honestly I did. Part of me didn't want to because I'm a pretty good judge of character but I don't think I signalled that in any way. I was positive, engaging, cheerful and open, and I launched into the detailed explanations and tried to get him involved in the conversation as often as possible. It was like pulling teeth. He would grunt, instead of answering questions, he would disagree with things that nobody normally disagreed with – things that weren't even worth disagreeing about, which made it obvious he was just being disagreeable. And all the time he surveyed me as if I was nothing but a liar and a charlatan. After about fifteen minutes, I had had enough. I felt like breaking his fat neck. And let's face it: you really do have to be a piece of work to get a *therapist* to feel like killing you. So I stopped short and asked him directly: "How do you feel your session is going, Duncan? Be honest!"

He looked at me scornfully, and said: "Well, to be frank I don't think you've said one thing so far that convinces me I should stop smoking!"

Aha. This guy actually thought it was my job to persuade people that they should stop smoking. So I enlightened him:

"You've got me all wrong, Duncan. It's not my job to convince you to stop! Clients are supposed to work that one out all by themselves before they come here. You see, here's how it works: people decide they don't want to smoke anymore, and then they decide *how* they are going to succeed in doing that. If they decide to use hypnotherapy, then they call me. You haven't even *begun* that process, so there is nothing for me to do here." Then I just gazed at him, until he figured out that the session was over all of a sudden. Even then, he couldn't quite believe it.

"What – is that *it*?"

"That's all there is to it!" I said in a light-hearted, matter-of-fact way.

"So you're not even going to do any... y'know, hypnosis?"

"No point."

This threw him completely. He wasn't expecting that. He thought he was in charge because that was what he was used to - and anyway he had me down as a fake - just interested in his money - and here I was turning him and his money away, voluntarily? That didn't fit in with his idea of what I was about. Why would I do that, when he would certainly have paid me for my time? Only to have the petty satisfaction of proving that hypnotherapy wouldn't 'work on' *him*, of course.

## A Refusal or a Failure to Respond

In reality, any idiot can fail to respond to hypnotherapy. You simply adopt a negative attitude to the process. This doesn't demonstrate that you have a strong mind, or a powerful independent will. You might have, but you certainly don't need to have that in order to waste the hypnotherapist's time. You can also do it by being so stupid you can't follow simple directions, being compulsively uncooperative, generally disagreeable or by simply not wishing to respond. Therefore: any idiot can do it.

Duncan had absolutely no inclination to be positive about anything I said, which is a position that any bad-tempered sod could adopt quite effortlessly. What really stunned him was the fact that I was effectively dismissing him. And so early on, too – he probably thought he could irritate me for the full session but now here he was with no real option but to get up out of the comfortable chair, put his jacket back on and leave. Not because he wanted to but because I had finished with him, and that made it uncomfortably obvious to him that in my office he had no authority at all. Evidently his money didn't count for anything either, which must be really confusing if you have someone down as a con-artist. Think again, buddy.

As he left, he was one very unhappy chappie. But then he was a miserable swine when he came in, so I didn't feel responsible for that. As he walked out, he said something very telling indeed: "I thought at least I might be able to *relax* for an hour or so!" In other words, he had no intention of stopping smoking at all. He didn't come to my office to work with me, but to be cocky and obstructive, and I was particularly unimpressed with that because his wife had been so much the reverse. What was she doing with a grumpy prat like him?

So I terminated that session abruptly rather than waste my breath, and of course I didn't charge for that one. Which may seem like just a financial loss, on the face of it... but oh, if you could have seen the look on that old misery's face as he realised I was effectively kicking him out – worth every penny. I treated myself to that one. I'm worth it.

Incidentally, if anyone ever tells you that they "don't suffer fools gladly" - as if they are *proud* of their judgemental intolerance – confuse them by saying cheerfully: "But the world's full of fools! How on earth do you cope?"

Personally, I quite like fools. Been one meself, numerous times! It's bullies I can't stand.

# Section Seventeen

## Hypnotherapy v. Science

## *or* The Myopia of the conscious mind (A Historical Perspective)

The history and development of the hypnotherapy profession is littered with lost opportunities, bad timing, persecuted pioneers, skepticism, general fear and prejudice and, above all, ignorance. In truth, the therapeutic use of trance and suggestion goes back thousands of years, but for most of that time it was always bound up with various forms of religion, and until quite recently not understood as a specifically mental phenomenon outside of that spiritual context. Trance and suggestion do play some part in many cults and religions but only in the same way as they can play a role in political movements and any other belief system. Still, it is only since the mid-eighteenth century that the history of hypnotherapy itself moves into the academic sphere and, like many subjects in that era, was generally misunderstood right from the beginning.

This is a brief sketch of a few significant moments in the history of hypnotherapy which I will begin with a very colourful character called Franz Anton Mesmer, a Viennese physician who believed he could cure illnesses using magnetism. Mesmer certainly misunderstood what he was actually doing but he wasn't a quack. In fact he was very successful, which so annoyed some of his medical colleagues that he was soon obliged to leave Vienna and set up a clinic in Paris. This quickly became one of the most famous clinics in Europe.

Mesmer was arguably the first significant "hypnotherapist", although he would not have recognised the term. He was the first to become internationally famous through consistently healing ailments using nothing but suggestion, yet with no religious or spiritual dimension to the process. It's just that he didn't know that suggestion was the key. He thought it was all brought about through some sort of healing magnetic flow of energy. He conceptualised this as an invisible fluid which he could personally direct, and in this respect the idea has similarities with the notion of *chi* in Chinese medicine, an energy flow. Elements of Reiki here too, with Mesmer conceiving of himself as a conduit of this energy personally, like a channeller, but (unlike Reiki) without any spiritual dimension to the concept. For Mesmer, it was an invisible aspect of Physics, and he called it Animal Magnetism.

Healing which involved magnetism was not Mesmer's innovation. He had been a student of a Viennese Jesuit named Father Maximilian Hell, who had been using magnets and steel plates to heal. These were apparently applied to the naked body. Yes, it sounds so soothing doesn't it? Sick and buck naked, having steel plates pressed against your trembling body by a man called Father Hell.

Prior to that, there was "The Great Irish Stroker" Valentine Greatrakes, famous for healing by passing his hands (and also magnets) over the body. But credited – if that is an appropriate term - as the first to use magnets in healing processes was the Swiss physician Paracelsus (1493-1541). He also developed a cure for syphilis involving mercury, which of course is highly poisonous. Yes, if you ever thought some modern alternative therapies were far-fetched, you should read up on the history of medicine. Anyway people were successfully cured, it seems, when Paracelsus passed magnets (or lodestones) over their body.

So there were precedents, but Mesmer went considerably further in terms of both style and invention, and brought a real sense of theatre to the business of healing. Somebody should make a movie about Mesmer, he was a real star. It was no wonder he was such a hit because not only did his methods work well for many people, they were exciting and even spectacular at times, for Mesmer was a true showman. Despite being essentially a doctor, he created quite a dramatic scene in his clinic. He would treat many people at the same time, mainly because of demand. He invented a piece of 'magnetising' equipment called a baquet, which was a large oak tub placed in the centre of the room. This was filled with water, iron filings and powdered glass (which was then believed to have magnetic properties), and jointed iron rods came up out of the water through holes in the lid. These could be grasped by patients sitting around the tub or held to the affected part of the body, which was then 'magnetised'.

But this was not a clinical setting as we would expect to encounter today. The windows were heavily curtained, and plaintive music was creating an emotional atmosphere. Then Mesmer himself would appear, dressed in lilac silken robes and holding a long iron wand. He went from patient to patient, 'magnetising' them either by passing his hands over their bodies, or with the wand. Sometimes he would fix his gaze directly upon their eyes.

This combination of extraordinary and mood-enhancing factors diverts the patient's attention away from the everyday world. Thus perceptions, thought and feelings are free to roam into the realm of the Imaginary, where just about anything is possible (to the mind), including 'miraculous' cures. The effect was quite literally mesmerising, which is of course the origin of the word. To put it simply, it is trance-inducing. This is not really as bizarre as it sounds because exactly the same effect can be created in many other contexts, such as a beautiful cathedral, with a good choir in full song. Or on the terraces of a big football game, just before a penalty kick in the last minute of the match. A similar experience can be felt in a casino, watching the roulette ball go round and round... and we may find ourselves in the same state in a movie theatre, if we are gripped by the action. But instead of becoming fascinated by flickering images on a screen, these people were fascinated by Mesmer. He *was* the movie, and when a person knows how to make that kind of impact, things happen.

Now the idea that he *made* things happen, personally, is both incorrect and yet oddly correct at the same time. Incorrect because it is actually suggestion which made the changes happen. Or to be more precise, the Subconscious response of Mesmer's patients to those suggestions - there is no power in a suggestion itself. So in the cases of all those who healed or improved the experience was real, it was just their understanding of it that was flawed. They thought Mesmer was healing the body directly by 'magnetising' it: influencing the energy flow throughout the body and thus re-balancing the natural state of health. Mesmer believed that himself - but just because he had the wrong impression of what was really happening doesn't mean he was a fraud. Something was happening all right but it was going to be many years before it was understood more accurately.

Even today – now that there are some of us who understand it very well because we work with these things all the time - two centuries after Mesmer the majority of people in the world still do not know that any of this is even possible, much less understand it. Yet hypnotherapists should not be too disheartened by that fact because this unnecessary persistence of ignorance doesn't only apply to the kind of work we do. When Nicolas Copernicus first published his theory that the Earth actually orbited the Sun, and not the other way round, it was over a century before *anyone at all* publicly recognised the truth of it. And even then, they had a hell of a job convincing everybody else.

So Mesmer was literally incorrect in his belief that he was personally doing the healing with magnetism. But who created the *suggestions* to which they genuinely responded? Mesmer! Who curtained the windows, chose the music, provided the equipment and all the rest of the theatrics, who dreamed up the lilac robes and the iron wand? Mesmer!

Actually, it would be more accurate to note that he simply borrowed all the theatrics from religion and the church. They had been using these trappings for centuries to create a sense of mystery, power and importance around themselves. If you want to end up with a worldwide flock of millions of believers, it's no good turning up in a T-shirt. It *has* to be robes, doesn't it? And some sort of special hat? And you've got to have a wand, or a staff of some sort - that's a must. What magician doesn't have something like that? And if you have a mental image of the Pope right now, you can see where Mesmer's inspiration was coming from.

I don't mean to offend anyone by drawing a parallel between a magician and a Pope, I am merely commenting upon the effect of appearance when it comes to suggestions of power. The last Pope is now being posthumously credited with performing a number of miracles whilst he was alive, and obviously the way he presented himself would have had to have been in keeping with the implications of that.

I don't know what casual garments Popes typically lounge around in, but if you consider ceremonial Papal attire it is obvious that if I wore an outfit like that to work, in my capacity as a modern hypnotherapist, most people would have doubts about me. I may be making assumptions but I don't think too many people would want to come to me for therapy – in fact they would probably conclude that I needed therapy myself. As indeed we all do from time to time, but the point is, when the Pope puts that gear on thousands flock from all over the world just to catch a glimpse of him. Do you think they would bother to do that if he just wore the sort of modest clothes I wear to the office? Well exactly, that's the kind of difference costume alone can make.

Mesmer knew. He wasn't a modern hypnotherapist, you see – he was a flamboyant pioneer, so he was aiming to make a big impression. And there's nothing quite like silken robes of lilac if you really want to be noticed.

For you see, if Mesmer hadn't done any of those things, his clinic would not have been anything like as famous at the time. And that very popularity, the buzz and the excitement surrounding him added to the impact of all the suggestion, creating more expectation and therefore more response. So although he didn't heal anyone directly, he did personally play a very significant role in the process that led to them healing themselves and they would not have managed to do that without his performance being a catalyst to the process. So he was - in effect, if not quite directly - a healer. He certainly wasn't a fraud.

But he must have looked like one to some, especially his enemies. The trouble with success and popularity is that it can lead to jealousy. Mesmer had his followers, but not everybody liked his style and eventually the King of France was persuaded to put together a Board of Inquiry to examine and test the validity of Mesmer's methods. This Board included several eminent scientists of the time: Benjamin Franklin, the chemist Lavoisier and a certain Doctor Guillotin. He is credited with being an expert in pain control, but he is most famous for inventing a machine that made pain control no longer necessary. Sometime later the French used it to remove their Head of State. The story goes that it took three attempts because his neck was so fat. A bad enough end for the Head of State, but the state of the neck was worse. So much for pain control Doc.

Anyway, these skeptical characters ended up refuting Mesmer's claims, which Franklin dismissed by saying: "If these people are healed at all, they are only healed in their imagination!" This is as close to the truth as you can get whilst still being entirely wrong.

## Imaginary Does Not Simply Mean Unreal

The concept of imagination that casts it as opposed to reality, or unconnected with it, is a fundamental error and a conceit of the conscious mind. Imagination is always directly connected with the real in one way or another – how could it not be? Inevitably, the activities of the imagination are a real reaction to the conditions of the external reality. Such imaginings could only have significance insofar as they relate to the external reality, obviously. In fact they have to do only with that, so imagination doesn't relate to anything *but* the real. Our ability to conceive of things *beyond* actual experience is an essential factor when it comes to *changing* reality, which humans are pretty good at. Long before mobile telecommunications could become a reality, for example, someone had to dream up the whole idea at a time when the notion was quite impossible in reality. As Leonardo knew when he was sketching his helicopter ideas five hundred years ago: reality changes. He was using his imagination, but there is nothing unreal about helicopters now.

Imagination is really just Subconscious thought. Everything that appeals to the imagination is appealing to the Subconscious. The Subconscious controls the body in every respect and to the finest detail. If we bring a problem in that arena to the attention of the Subconscious and make a useful suggestion, the Subconscious mind is then in a position to attend to it, whether it actually chooses to do so or not. Whether a placebo is involved in the process or anyone believes magnetism is involved, or crystals, or *chi,* or fairy dust is neither here nor there.

Let me backtrack a little. I do not mean to *insist* that none of those things have any useful essence of their own, only that they need none to function in that way. The placebo effect is nothing more or less than the response of the Subconscious to suggestion. With placebo 'medications' we know that it cannot be anything else because the substance is inert – it does nothing - but a prerequisite in that part of the individual's belief system is the suggestion that Science can help you, that doctors and their medicines can make you better. This may not elicit such a powerful response – or any response - in a person who has always held that all doctors are quacks. But if the same person grew up surrounded by folk who swore that if The Great Irish Stroker ever laid his marvellous hands upon you, all sickness will leave your body – yea, they are like the healing hands of Jesus Christ himself! - well that is a different matter. Beliefs play quite an important role in all this.

## After Mesmer

Mesmer then retired to Switzerland, probably thinking "I don't know why I bother!" Trance phenomena quickly made a comeback though, round about the time of Mesmer's death in 1815, when an Indo-Portuguese priest called Abbe Faria started doing demonstrations in Paris, only without the magnetising equipment. Faria held the view that the effect came from within the mind, and that expectancy and co-operation were key elements in obtaining good results. He was right, and this brought the process a step closer to what we now call hypnotherapy. His work was later developed by Bernheim and Liebault of the French Nancy School.

Before any of this ever became known as 'hypnosis' two other 'firsts' occurred. A student of Mesmer's called the Marquis de Puysegur described a profound state of trance and named it "somnambulism". His followers still believed in the theory of a magnetic fluid, and they called themselves Experimentalists. Then in 1821, a pioneering surgeon by the name of Recamier was the first to operate on patients who were in a mesmeric state. This was before chemical anaesthetics were discovered, and it represented the first major opportunity for the medical profession to realize that:

> "The potential for mind-body medicine is enormous,"

...as John Gruzelier, Professor of Psychology at Imperial College London said excitedly in 2002, a mere 181 years later. What is really quite difficult to understand is why medical authorities seem to have been so determined during the last couple of centuries to reject, ignore or deny the validity of all the exciting developments that followed at regular intervals, right up to the present day. If we recall what Professor Michael Baum et al. said in 2006, in their refutation of the use of alternative therapies within the NHS:

> "...our ability to explain and justify to patients the selection of treatments, and to account for expenditure on them more widely, is compromised if we abandon our reference to evidence."

...we have to wonder why such persons within the medical establishment have seen fit to pointedly ignore almost all the evidence relating to hypnosis that has emerged during the last seven generations. I will run through the main parts briefly here, just to give you some idea.

Following Recamier's success in 1821 with mesmeric anaesthesia in surgery, which I think every normal person would agree was an exciting development, Carl Reichenbach ran scientific studies throughout the 1840s and 1850s to test the validity of 'mesmeric energy', which he called Odic Force. The Force may have been with him, but the rest of the scientific community rejected his conclusions, entirely on the basis that Mesmer had already been denounced. They simply did not want any of it to turn out to be genuine because that would suggest that the mainstream view was incorrect... and that state of affairs has more or less persisted to this day.

Throughout the middle of the 19th Century there appears to have been great controversy about anything to do with mesmerism or animal magnetism within the British medical establishment, and views were polarising – if you will forgive the pun. This may have been because Mesmer had been quite a colourful figure himself *and* that he had been officially declared a fraud, or perhaps because of the early emphasis on magnetism, which seemed obviously a mistake anyway. Either way the establishment quickly took up the position that mesmerism was quackery and should be stamped out. For quite a while, surgery was the main battleground - for one could not call this a debate. What is really striking about the disagreements in the mid- to late-nineteenth century between medics is how hostile and abusive they became. These were not cool-headed, analytical scientific investigations into the truth of this or that. No, these were highly emotional exchanges, and in considering these bad-tempered conflicts I am reminded of that psychologist and her smoking session at my office. Her hostility, her bitter resentment towards NLP and hypnosis really had nothing to do with smoking, it was all about career and reputation, professional standing and the threat posed to all of that by the success of other methods like NLP.

There was a battle going on for the soul of the medical profession two centuries ago, and three major figures in the pre-history of the hypnotherapy profession were at the centre of it. Of these, the most brilliant was Dr John Elliotson (1791-1868), President of the Royal Medical and Surgical Society and one of the Founders of University College Hospital, London, where he became its first Professor of Medicine. He made his reputation in the 1830s giving public lectures on various aspects of medicine and many of these lectures were published in the Lancet. In 1837 he became interested in the work of the Baron du Potet, a successful mesmerist who was visiting London at the time.

Elliotson was no fool. He is credited with introducing the stethoscope to England, and narcotics, both from France where he had studied. He developed methods of examining the heart and lungs which are still in use today. He was quick to realise the potential of mesmerism for achieving conditions for painless surgery, and through his own experiments at University College Hospital soon proved the value of mesmeric states in the treatment of nervous disorders as well as other medical cases. But it was the anaesthetic aspects of mesmerism that were the most immediately exciting in those early days of surgery, before ether and chloroform were discovered.

Now you might assume that medical people – intelligent, educated men, after all – would be very interested in these developments, for which the applications are obvious and potentially advantageous to the profession as a whole. Perhaps Mesmer had been too readily dismissed and there might be something useful there after all? You would expect, at the very least, that the skeptics would be able to control themselves enough to be civilised about the public demonstrations, and the experiments that should surely follow so that whatever good that might come of this method could be successfully arrived at, for the benefit of all.

You would be wrong. Never underestimate the power of professional envy and jealousy to distort human judgement and temper, as this extract from the Lancet shows (1842):

> The patient, alias the victim, alias the *particeps criminis,* is almost as bad as the operator; and even the man who reads about such performances, is a leper.

Close friends of Elliotson at the time of his public demonstrations of mesmerism were Charles Dickens and William Thackery, which I guess makes them lepers too. Elliotson taught Dickens how to use mesmerism to soothe his wife, who was a hypochondriac.

## The 'Spiritual' Angle

One aspect of all this which may have made Elliotson an easy target for his enemies was that he demonstrated how some of his patients apparently became 'clairvoyant' whilst in mesmeric trance, and sometimes made diagnoses. Not everybody who works with hypnosis professionally will be inclined to take this 'extra-sensory' aspect of trance states seriously - and even some of those that are may be reluctant to speak of such things openly for fear of becoming the next David Icke in the eyes of more skeptical people. Actually I think that this can be avoided by keeping an open mind and a sense of humour about these things, but I do think that to notice curious phenomena and yet to never speak of them is actually just cowardice. Of course cowardice has always been commonplace enough and is entirely understandable, since one would not expect anyone who has not personally experienced curiosities of this nature on a regular basis to believe a word of it, especially if they are not open-minded about such matters in the first place.

Some were. Dr James Esdaile (1805-1859), a young Scottish surgeon, was inspired by Elliotson's teaching to perform hundreds of operations upon mesmerised patients. He also wrote a book called *Natural and Mesmeric Clairvoyance* in which he referred to this aspect of Elliotson's work. For some, this was taking matters in a non-scientific direction and both Esdaile and Elliotson were about to discover that, for the time being at least, the battle for the soul of the medical profession was not going to be won by anyone who was open-minded about things like clairvoyance, but by the bullying, cynical, mocking element who did not believe that the profession *had* a soul. Or indeed that anyone had, for that matter.

The board of Trustees at University College Hospital asked Elliotson to stop putting on public displays of mesmerism, and in 1838 the Council of the University passed a resolution forbidding the use of mesmerism in the hospital. Elliotson immediately resigned. The Dean of the University tried to persuade him to give up mesmerism so that he could retain his position in the hospital. Elliotson replied that the University which he had co-founded "was established for the discovery and dissemination of truth. All other considerations are secondary. We should lead the public, not the public us. The sole question is whether the matter is the truth or not."

Now think back, all you open-minded readers, to the various quotes I have assembled and presented throughout this book from modern scientific and medical sources who keep repeating the mantra that there is "no evidence" of success using hypnotherapy and other alternative approaches, or that "many systematic reviews have failed to find..." etc. This is either sheer ignorance, or it is dissembling and denial. The truth is that it never was a lack of evidence that was the problem even two centuries ago, but a lack of tolerance, objectivity and vision. It is primarily the myopia of the conscious mind that has always been driving the denial of the realities of these things, combined with intellectual dogmatism, professional jealousy and plain old mean self-interest. These remain the factors that have prevented institutional acceptance of new ideas, or slowed it to a glacial crawl.

Elliotson couldn't abide the hypocrisy. He continued to use mesmerism and in 1843 he began publishing *Zoist,* a quarterly journal which recorded case after case of successful treatment. No scientific research to support the effectiveness of these methods? What a damned lie, it has been going on for generations ever since, it is just that the medical authorities in the Western world have been largely pretending it hasn't. The medical profession did not reject mesmerism and hypnosis because those methods were useless or unsuccessful, but because the brilliant, bright new thinkers were in the minority and the cowardly, dull-witted skeptics felt threatened by them. And – quite possibly – because of the mention of things like clairvoyance, which makes anyone an easy target for scorn and derision in the scientific world.

## Credo

You may be wondering what my own view of all that spiritual stuff may be. Well, in the ordinary course of my working day zero clairvoyance is involved. I don't even know if my clients are going to turn up, that's how clairvoyant I am. I believe in hypnotherapy because I happen to be particularly good at it and the results I get are frequently excellent and sometimes even amazing. There is nothing miraculous or paranormal about any of that though.

If someone else is doing the same thing but with a belief-system that included a spiritual angle, might they attribute some of that success to spiritual guidance or clairvoyance? Very possibly, and then the beneficial results they are able to bring about might seem to suggest that they must be right – but just like Mesmer, they may be doing the right sort of thing but completely misunderstanding exactly why it works.

Or possibly I may be wrong about there being no spiritual angle, in which case my spirit guides must be endlessly frustrated that I keep wrongly interpreting their celestial assistance as my own personal brilliance! Who knows?

## Back to the History

Later, as drug companies became more and more influential it just became easier for them and their lackeys to stamp out the calls for more non-drug therapies within the medical world by the sheer bullying weight of that industry's lobbying power. Nowadays the problem is institutional rather than intellectual - and to be fair to the medical profession as a whole, it is worth pointing out that this kind of ideological struggle can occur in any institution, it is not particular to them. It effectively becomes a war, and the first casualty of any war is of course truth.

Elliotson simply abandoned that institution, and instead he founded the Mesmeric Hospital in London in 1846, and others appeared in major cities including Edinburgh and Dublin. It was subsequently reported that in one such establishment in Exeter, a surgeon by the name of Dr Parker performed over two hundred successful operations using mesmerism. No, there never was any shortage of demonstration or evidence - it was just that the battle for control of medical orthodoxy was never about truth, but power, money and influence. It still is.

Despite his departure from the scientific mainstream and his insistence on continuing, and indeed expanding his work with mesmerism, John Elliotson was considered such an outstanding doctor that the Royal College of Physicians invited him to deliver the annual Harverian Lecture in 1846, the same year he founded the Mesmeric Hospital. His oration criticised Science for failing to seriously consider new ways of thinking, and naturally this further incensed his critics.

Another major figure who emerged during this extraordinary period was James Braid (1795-1860), who is now often referred to as the Father of Modern Hypnotism. Quite why Hypnotism should need a father figure is beyond me but people will tend to pin that sort of acolade on someone, so it went to him. He did develop eye-fixation induction techniques and also coined the term "hypnosis" - so that might have something to do with it – but true to the general confusion around the development of the art, this word is a misnomer. At the time, Braid surmised that certain parts of the brain became exhausted by gazing at a bright object until the eyes became tired, inducing "nervous sleep". First terming this *neuro-hypnosis,* he then shortened this to hypnosis (hypnos being a Greek word for sleep). At some point he realised there is no sleep in hypnosis and tried to amend this to *monoideism,* but snappy though that was, it didn't catch on and we have been stuck with the daft term 'hypnosis' ever since. If there was any way we could get rid of it, I think it would be a wonderfully liberating thing for the profession, but I'm not expecting that to occur anytime soon.

Braid's useful methods caught on however - even though his new term for it didn't - and other doctors reported success including an account published in 1842 describing an amputation without pain under hypnosis. This report was of course widely dismissed amongst the scientific community, who thenceforward proved themselves consistently content to abandon all reference to evidence wherever hypnosis was concerned. Note how these negative reactions are not happening because the methods didn't work, but because the people on the other side simply didn't want these methods to be used, or their proponents to be professionally more successful than them. It was really just a battle for influence within the medical establishment, and the skeptics won because skepticism is easy. It requires no vision, insight, talent or uncommon intelligence. Any fool can manage to produce knee-jerk reactions of scorn and derision, and inevitably many of these people turned out to be the old guard in the influential positions who were obviously content with the status quo, and their up-and-coming proteges.

It is also observable that ambitious types with less real talent tend to claw their way to the top politically, through toadying within the Institution – a creepy process that would have been completely alien to men like Elliotson or Braid. Behind closed doors, and in the corridors of power such sluggards may conspire against those who should reach the highest positions of influence through sheer brilliance, and in various fields – not just medicine – many a true star has been done down by the weasely competition in exactly this way, more's the pity.

Meanwhile in India, James Esdaile was establishing a reputation for success with mesmerism in surgery during 1845, and after a government committee reported favourably upon his work he was placed in charge of a special hospital in Calcutta in 1846. Here he performed several thousand minor and around three hundred major surgical procedures using mesmeric states as the only form of anaesthesia. In those early days in the development of modern surgery patients often died on the operating table, either through shock or loss of blood, but Esdaile succeeded in reducing the fatality rate from 50% to 5% with the use of mesmerism.

## An Aside

The common mythical notion that "some people can't be hypnotized" is effectively disproven by operators like Esdaile, and what this demonstrates is that we can work with anyone who is keen to benefit from the proceedings, whereas the Stage Hypnotist will encounter far more resistance and can only work with those who don't mind being in the show – which is the source of the myth, of course, because that rules most people out. How many people would like to feel no pain during surgery? Everyone, correct. So it is not 'hypnosis' that some people resist, but certain types of suggestion.

## Back to Esdaile's Phenomenal Success

Again, it has to be said that any normal person should regard Esdaile's achievements as very exciting and encouraging. However, the Calcutta Medical College did its best to discredit him, even spreading the rumour that his patients, who had undergone major operations without pain, were "a set of hardened and determined imposters", which we have to regard as resorting to a jaw-droppingly desperate suggestion. Initially, these attacks turned opinion against Esdaile and he was attacked by local newspapers. But following case after case of painless surgery, involving thousands of people, press opinion reversed and they turned on the orthodox medical authorities who had tried to mislead them.

Encouraged by this success Esdaile returned to England to present his findings to the medical authorities. He kept meticulous records of all his work, which included major operations such as amputations, removal of tumours, deep abdominal surgery and even eyeball removal – all carried out with mesmerism as the only anaesthetic. In each case there was no apparent pain or distress, and there were very few fatalities. He probably hoped his work would be greeted with great excitement. He couldn't have been more wrong. The medical journals flatly refused to print details of his pain-free operations using mesmerism, claiming – of all things – that they were "unpractical", thus completely abandoning all reference to the actual *evidence,* Professor Baum, in a way that amounts to putting their hands over their ears, shutting their eyes and humming loudly. This excerpt from the Lancet sums up the attitude of the medical authorities at the time:

> Mesmerism is too gross a humbug to admit of any further serious notice. We regard its abettors as quacks and imposters. They ought to be hooted out of professional Society. Any practitioner who sends a patient afflicted with any disease to consult a mesmeric quack, ought to be without patients for the rest of his days.

James Esdaile was ordered by the medical authorities to cease his work using mesmerism. After considering his findings, they concluded that the experience of pain was by God's Design, and that to remove it was to meddle with the Will of God. Esdaile returned to India, probably thinking "I don't know why I bother!" and continued flouting the will of God, or to be more precise the medical authorities. Soon after this, the discovery of ether and later chloroform led to the highly unusual occurrence of God Changing His Will.

The passing of these three medical heroes of hypnotism marked the end of surgical applications for quite a while, mainly because any fool can pour out a measured quantity of ether or chloroform, without having to understand the human mind at all, and just knock it out – or at least, the conscious bit. It was the chemical equivalent of a mallet, and of course it had its risks, unlike hypnosis or mesmerism which have never been known to have any real risks associated with them, only imaginary ones.

## Later Brief Applications of Hypnosis

Hypnosis was used a good deal by field doctors in the American Civil War (1861-1865), and this was the first truly extensive medical use of the method, but again it was short-lived because of the invention of the hypodermic needle and chemical anaesthesia. It made something of a comeback during World War I in the treatment of "shell-shock", and was also used in a number of subsequent wars as a technique within the field of psychiatry to address the problem of what is now termed "post-traumatic stress disorder".

Was that hypnotherapy, though? Well, yes and no. Yes, because it obviously involves the use of trance states in an attempt to restore mental and physical well-being. No, because psychiatrists were doing it and hypnotherapy was not their profession. Surely these people spent many years studying psychiatry, not hypnotherapy. Their training in the use of hypnosis would have been so cursory that they were, in effect, dabblers.

This does not prevent them from being perfectly capable of using that technique to deal with that particular issue, but once they became qualified psychiatrists, how much of their professional time did they spend actually using hypnotherapy? Probably very little - and mainly within these narrow military applications, just treating battle-related disorders mostly.

This sort of limited application does not result in a deep and broad understanding of the field of hypnotherapy, but simply produces a psychiatrist with a useful technique for treating traumatised survivors of terrifying conflict. Such an operator would have little or no practical knowledge of the usefulness of hypnotherapy outside of that - very little awareness of what else the Subconscious is capable of changing. They would also have no experience at all of working with people who were not ill or traumatised, which would actually be a fair description of the majority of my clients, since I am not a psychiatrist. I am generally working with people who are fine, actually – they just want to change something.

As a professional hypnotherapist, I spend between 30 and 40 hours every week doing hypnotherapy and nothing else... which means that I already have well over seventeen thousand hours of practical experience in the art of hypnotherapy, working with thousands of different individuals who present with all manner of issues. That is a different order of experience altogether. Do you see my point? Whatever professional knowledge those psychiatrists may have possessed, very little of it was about hypnosis in reality. But now it is time to return to the historical progression of the "knowledge" as it fared outside the field of military conflict, as hypnosis had one of its many revivals in popularity towards the end of the nineteenth century. This was due to new scientific interest in how the mind itself actually worked and the study of mental illness and instability, or dysfunction.

## Enter: The Head-Doctors

So now the baton passed to the neurologists and those developing the mind-sciences, such as Charcot and Freud. Much has been written about them so I don't need to re-hash any of that, but it is worth noting that during this phase in the history of hypnosis-as-therapy, the emphasis is on work done with patients who were suffering from 'hysteria' or 'neuroses' of one sort or another. Today there is no such illness as 'hysteria' but it was reckoned to be all too common at the time. What is glaringly obvious nowadays is that the characters at the centre of these investigations were seriously misunderstanding the conditions they were trying to treat *as well as* the methods they were attempting to use, which was not really the case with the earlier surgeons. Consequently their successes were rarely as dramatic.

Still, certain new aspects of hypnotic phenomena were discovered during this phase, including regression, dissociation and post-hypnotic suggestion. Liebault pointed out the importance of rapport: the trust relationship between the 'hypnotizer' and the 'hypnotized'. Various theories of suggestibility were proposed, as well as 'Laws' of suggestion. These were really just observations, and cannot be regarded as truly established laws such as we assume the laws of physics to be, by contrast, when they are first presented to us. As Scotty said: "Ye cannae change the laws of physics, Jim!" This has never been the case when it comes to suggestion.

Hypnotherapy as a profession did not exist during all of these developments. These people were never hypnotherapists, they were doctors and scientists experimenting with hypnotic procedures that they did not understand very well at all, using them *as techniques* in the treatment of mental problems they misunderstood anyway. This haphazard and limited application resulted in limited success and limited understanding, as well as a good deal of misunderstanding.

As a result, the temporary use of hypnosis in the aftermath of the various wars that followed was such a specific and short-term application that it was never going to bring hypnotherapy into the medical mainstream. Since then its use in modern Western medicine has been negligible – not because of any lack of potential application but because of the colossal influence of the drug industry which fiercely defends its territory against all alternative therapies via the conservative hierarchy in the medical authority structures. In fact I would posit that at this point in history, Western medical science belongs to the pharmaceutical industry, the two are indistinguishable. It is big business posing as healthcare. Of course they don't want a fit and healthy population, it would be bad for business, wouldn't it?

## Hypnotherapy is Not Medicine

Ironically, hypnotherapy has truly thrived outside the medical profession and the understanding of the art has come on in leaps and bounds during the last two or three generations – possibly because it has been free to develop quite naturally. There are institutions within the profession but not one of them has exclusive control, so they have a light regulatory touch. This is nevertheless safe enough because hypnotherapy is a process which can only have a practical outcome or no outcome. This is because the results are not governed by the therapist but by the individual client's preferred response to the verbal presentation, which makes it more akin to education than medicine. To call it "treatment" is really a bit of a misunderstanding.

## Real Hypnotherapy: The Growth of an Invisible Art

Lay (as in non-medical) practitioners of hypnotherapy were probably quietly growing in numbers from the end of the nineteenth century, partly because there was a general popular interest in all areas of scientific development. Freud's published work was quite widely read, and just as ordinary individuals might become fascinated by things like photography, railway engines and other aspects of science and engineering, so some people picked up on mesmerism and hypnosis. However, these people – the real enthusiasts - are more or less invisible in the official, literary history of hypnosis, because histories are compiled by academics and inevitably tend to be the history of academia, or to be more precise, a selective history of academic publishing on the subject. And so we come to:

## The Psychologists

The modern academic study of hypnotism is reputed to have begun in the 1930s with the work of an experimental psychologist called Clark Hull, who used statistical and experimental analysis at Yale University to carry out extensive research resulting in the publication of *Hypnosis and Suggestibility* in 1933. This began a series of investigations into the characteristics of trance states, the majority of which were carried out in an analytical manner, where the attempt was to define what can and what apparently cannot be done with hypnosis. I say 'apparently', because if a researcher can produce an effect, then that certainly proves it can be done. But if a researcher cannot achieve something with the application of a hypnotic 'technique', that certainly does not prove that it cannot be achieved by the use of hypnosis. A newly-qualified pilot with limited flying experience cannot produce a dazzling display of daring aerobatics, but that doesn't mean it cannot be done. What you need for that is an expert with a great deal of practical experience, and the problem with nearly all the publishing and research in the mind-sciences regarding hypnosis as a therapeutic tool is that it was unheard-of for any professional hypnotherapists to be involved in it. Consequently it reads, to the expert hypnotherapist, rather like the alchemist's methods would read to the modern chemist. Sometimes we don't know whether to laugh or cry.

So I am not going to review any of that research, nor list here the 'key' publications that followed because the vast majority of it is far less useful and inspiring than the original, hands-on work that was done by men like Elliotson and Esdaile. Professional hypnotherapists – especially the really good ones – have far more in common with the surgeons than the psychologists because the attitude we share is: Let's fix that. Now. And if we can work out a quicker or more effective way, let's adopt that. The methods are not theories, but practical applications that must prove themselves in regular successes, otherwise they will be dropped. We are not aiming to make slow or gradual improvements. Talented surgeons and talented hypnotherapists both aim for immediate and total success wherever possible, but psychologists do not expect that sort of change to result from *their* methods, so they have to convince themselves that the dramatic successes of hypnotherapy are hype, or else the whole field of psychology as a science would implode.

This need within the psychology field to avoid or undermine hypnosis therefore has to be taken into account when considering any 'research' involving hypnosis which has been published in that field in the last couple of generations, as Psychology has struggled to assert itself as a valid science. Not all of that research is worthless, obviously, but Psychology has been so afraid of not being taken seriously as a 'true science' that it has been effectively hamstrung by its own self-doubt: this is a neurosis within the field itself. The psychologists know what the medical authorities did to the mesmerists, and they are well aware that the mighty Freud abandoned the use of hypnosis early on. This makes any investigations into hypnosis politically dangerous territory within the scientific world – a bit like studying telepathy or telekinesis. If you are going to risk doing it at all, you had better make those studies super-skeptical and cautious in the extreme or your reputation will be ripped to shreds in the critical backlash, especially if you actually discover something interesting.

Above all, if you are going to risk publishing studies that involve hypnosis at all, you must never get excited or ambitious - that would just be foolhardy because in the scientific world such energy and liveliness is regarded as giddy and improper. No, let disbelief and low expectations be your constant companions - and if you do encounter any exciting developments, see if you can't think up a few possible complications that might explain them away, or at least cast doubt upon them yourself before anyone else does. And of course you must end your tentative (in)conclusions with the scientific mantra "More research is needed."

How many truly great advances in medical science resulted from that kind of paranoid hedging? It is precisely because hypnotherapists never have to bother with all that nonsense that we have developed so rapidly, but psychologists dare not recognise that as a fact without admitting that sacrificing hypnosis on the altar of analytical conscious skepticism just to beg for a place at the High Table of Science was a mistake in the first place.

## What Psychology merely labels, Hypnotherapy Fixes

Being unable to work with the Subconscious because of conscious limitations, fear and denial is a serious shortcoming in psychology, the medical profession and the scientific community at large. The pity is that the longer this continues – and it has already been the case for almost two centuries – the longer many people will be unaware that safe, effective and rapid solutions already exist for conditions and troubles they are being wrongly advised cannot be easily resolved, and for which they are often given medications that do not cure them. This is the LIE at the centre of the belief that hypnotherapy is:

> "...too gross a humbug to admit of any further serious notice."

It wasn't true then, and it isn't true now. Medics, scientists, psychologists – whatever - examine your consciences. Of course I am not addressing those that do not have consciences, for they will be what they are and I did not write any of this expecting to change their leaden opinions or their self-serving natures. They are the problem, just as they were two hundred years ago and it is probably impossible for them to ever form part of the solution.

## New Institutions

Elliotson had the right idea. Those who admire his spirit and find his legacy inspiring should follow his example. Instead of trying to get alternative therapies grudgingly accepted into the NHS, what is needed is a New Health Organisation quite outside the existing institutions. An Organisation that actually promotes health - instead of attempting to medicate the entire population – and helps people to liberate themselves from the bad habits and unhealthy lifestyles that cause ill-health in the first place. And not just by lecturing them, but by providing therapeutic assistance that actually works for the majority. Starting on a small and local scale, I suggest that the keen, bright and open-minded health professionals of the future who want to work with people, not diseases, abandon the old institutions and create a new project, taking the best each culture has to offer in the development of a natural approach to health and well-being that has nothing to do with the drug companies and simply exists as separate from those industries.

Then let people choose freely whether they prefer to spend years taking medications that don't cure them, with the occasional glimpse of a consultant who spends far more time and effort working on improving his golf swing than trying to improve their condition, or have someone like myself spend hours actively helping them. Let the NHS stumble on as it is, for as long as it can. We need not concern ourselves with that, nor seek to undermine it. Let's just move on – and be sure to take with us the spirit of those dynamic pioneers that went before. Let them at last be honoured - not by pomp, which they would not have appreciated anyway I'm sure – but by following their example. As Elliotson noted, we need only concern ourselves with:

> "...the discovery and dissemination of truth. All other considerations are secondary. We should lead the public, not the public us. The sole question is whether the matter is the truth or not."

## Case Mysteries 10: Mysterious Disappearances

Q: What is the number one cause of failure in hypnotherapy sessions?

A: The client not turning up!

The irony is that some of those who fail to turn up are probably dissuaded by a fear of failure. So they get cold feet - thus turning the mere outside possibility of failure into an absolute certainty.

Of all the appointments entered in my diary, I know that about a quarter of them will not happen on that day, or will never happen at all. And since most of those people would actually have been successful, that's a bit of a shame. Yet we have to accept the inevitability of this and seek to understand it rather than condemn. People get scared. They think of all their previous attempts to succeed with other methods and fill themselves with doubt and negativity, lose the impetus that made them book the session, wrongly assume that the hypnotherapy method will be no more successful than any of their previous attempts and then find that they just can't face it.

Sometimes people are astonished when I talk about the number of people who cancel at the last minute, postpone or just fail to arrive. They often comment that it's a terrible way to behave and expect me to be very annoyed about it. One or two of them even get annoyed about it on my behalf, and are then confused by the fact that I don't join in. Of course it is easy to look at it that way but as a keen student of the human mind I am more interested in the actual reasons for it than in judging people or getting all resentful.

## I've Changed!

Of course when I was starting out and I hardly had any bookings, I was excited when someone arranged to have hypnotherapy and I looked forward to the session. So the first time a client didn't show up and I got no phone call to explain why, I was understandably quite cross. It represented a real financial loss for one thing, especially when you hardly have any clients to begin with, but also I thought it was rude and inconsiderate to simply not turn up. So I rang the lady concerned, and she explained that the reason for her non-arrival was that she had bumped her car that very morning, so could she come next week instead? I was very relieved that I hadn't lost a client after all... until the following week when she failed to turn up for that one as well.

Bumped her car, eh? Yes, it is truly astonishing how many cars get bumped, break down or fail to start on the very morning that the owner is booked in to stop smoking, drinking or gambling. Likewise it is so uncanny how many people's fathers, mothers or young children are taken into hospital, fall down stairs or are struck down with appendicitis or some such sudden illness when their loving relative was just about to become a happier and healthier person, that I have often wondered if there could be some malign, demonic force at work here.

Or perhaps they are just lying to me.

Because if these people were not lying, folks, you would expect to see the same level of misfortune affecting people booked in for all the other issues we deal with in hypnotherapy: weight loss, phobias, depression, pain relief, emotional issues or simple habits like nail biting:

"Oh, hi, it's Laura here, I've got an appointment with you tomorrow to stop biting my nails... but the thing is, my father fell down the stairs yesterday, and he's in intensive care, and mum's got no other means of visiting, only me driving her, because she's too disabled to use public transport, so I'm afraid I'll have to cancel the session tomorrow and get back to you when I know how long my father's going to be in for..."

Never happens. But if you swap "biting my nails" for "smoking", then it happens with amazing regularity. And yet, in handling these calls it is very important for me to be polite, concerned and reassuring:

"No, no, you go ahead and take care of those things, don't give it a second thought! Thanks for letting me know, I'll leave it with you. Just get back to me when things are back to normal."

Why should I be like that when I know people are lying to me? Well, for two reasons: firstly, even if this particular cancellation is a real inconvenience to me, it is most unprofessional to let that show. The client's feelings are paramount because this client may be back later, and they are going to remember how I handled this. Even if I never meet them in the end, I still don't want to upset them anyway because they might then say negative things about me to other people. And, most importantly, whilst I am sure that most of these accidents and emergencies are fictional it is Sod's Law that if I ever actually said:

> "Oh, for God's sake cut the crap! Do you think I'm an idiot? You've just got a hangover or something - just be honest and spare me all this garbage about your daft old dad falling down the stairs!"

...that would be the one time it would turn out to be true, wouldn't it? And that would be me shouting at a person whose father had genuinely had a dreadful accident and was now on a life-support machine, vital signs flickering. So, even if the chances of it being true are about one in a hundred, it just isn't worth the risk, is it?

There is another dimension too, which is worth bearing in mind. Oftentimes I may be fairly sure the reason I've been given isn't the real story but that does not necessarily mean that the real story is any less valid a reason to postpone, it might just be something they don't feel like sharing with me:

"Oh hi, is that the hypnotherapy man? Yes I was supposed to come in this morning to stop smoking, but the thing is, I met this incredible bloke, and he came back to my house last night and stayed over, and I've had hardly any sleep at all, and to be honest

I just feel much more like spending all day in bed with him, and eating lots of ice cream, rather than stopping smoking today! Is it OK to re-book for another time?"

Of course it is, sorry to hear about your car breaking down. Some things we can't do anything about, we just have to work around them. I'll leave it with you, then, I hope everything goes OK with the repairs...

The truth is, if someone ever was that honest with me I would not be remotely upset - how could you be? And we cannot expect people to share their real private events with us over the phone when all they want to do is cancel an arrangement, so really there is no need to be upset about this aspect of providing therapy services. Yes, at first the no-shows get you down. Some hypnotherapy trainers even suggest that we should charge for missed appointments, and perhaps there are readers amongst you who might feel inclined to agree with this. But it is unworkable! What are you going to do about it if the person refuses to pay? Sue them? Send the boys round?

> "We're here to give you a friendly warning. You've upset Big Al. He is one hypnotherapist you do not want to cross, trust me. I heard that you arranged a meet with Big Al, but then you never showed. That is not clever, not clever my friend. You'd better pay up, or your smart little hatchback here might be involved in a bit of an *accident,* and we wouldn't want that, now would we?"

It's ridiculous, isn't it? It strikes the wrong note entirely: the other, menacing side of therapy! It would make an arresting advert though:

> "If you turn up, we'll help you with your problem. But if you don't turn up, we'll come round and solve all your problems in one go, know what I mean?"

No, I decided long ago to simply adjust to the reality. The bookings in the diary are theoretical. They might happen, but not all of them will. Once you get used to that idea, you can be very flexible about it. At some point in time I stopped taking breaks, stopped taking lunch-hours. I just booked in sessions back to back. When everyone turns up, that makes for a demanding day but it is very productive for the practice. But then when someone postpones or doesn't show up, I get an unexpected break and that means my reaction is usually: "Great, now I can do some writing/have lunch/get my hair cut/go to the bank" or whatever, which I never have time to do otherwise. And as I mentioned in the Acknowledgements in Volume I, this book would not exist at all if it were not for the no-shows, so it does prove that every cloud has a silver lining after all.

In addition to all of that, it means I can always handle cancellations graciously because part of me is genuinely glad it has occurred. Thus trust and rapport can be maintained and any later sessions with that person are likely to go well.

### The End

*Oh! Is that it, then?*

Well, what more do you want?

*Dunno. It just seemed a bit of a lame ending, after all that controversial stuff earlier on.*

Go back and read that again, then.

*OK. But I still think you need a better ending.*

Such as?

*Well, something which rounds it off nicely, you know. That ending is too ordinary, like you just came to a halt.*

I do see your point. OK, let's add this last thought for the reader:

If you have never experienced success with hypnotherapy for yourself, it is most likely to be because you have never had hypnotherapy at all. Most people alive today have never even seriously considered the hypnotherapy approach to solving their problems and yet many of them will have some sort of an opinion about it. That's a bit like reviewing a restaurant you have never been to yourself.

When I first qualified to practice hypnotherapy, I called my father and said: "Dad, I'm now a qualified hypnotherapist. Tell your friends!" to which my father replied "Oh, I don't think I know anyone who would benefit from hypnotherapy." I said: "Dad, I really don't know anyone that wouldn't."

What do you think? Will that do?

*Well, it's an improvement. But there's still room for a bit more improvement if you ask me.*

My philosophy exactly.

# Appendix

The first Volume of this book was originally published in October 2007 and this second Volume was supposed to appear the following year because most of it was already written. However, as it always takes me ages to get around to finishing things like this, it took a bit longer. Just in case you might be curious as to what was in Volume I, here is a list of the Contents:

## Nicotine: The Drug That Never Was
## Volume I: The Biggest Medical Mistake of the 20<sup>th</sup> Century

Acknowledgements
Anecdote
Are You Trying to Tell Me How to Read?

**Section One**
The Emperor's New Clothes
The Biggest Medical Mistake of the 20<sup>th</sup> Century
Welcome, Skeptics!

**Section Two**
Stage Hypnosis (The Shorter Explanation)
A note on Paul McKenna
Case Mysteries No.1

**Section Three**
Cravings are Not Withdrawal Symptoms
Case Mysteries No.2

**Section Four**
Introducing: The Subconscious Mind
Case Mysteries No.3

**Section Five**
Why the Nicotine Addiction Theory is Wrong
Case Mysteries No.4

**Section Six**
Trance and Suggestion:
a). What Really Happens in a Hypnotherapy Session
b). The Role of Suggestion: How and Why We Respond

**Section Seven**
Why Nicotine is not even a Drug
*also* The Inhalation of Smoke
& Rattus Humanus

**Section Eight**
What Cravings Really Are, and How we Shut them Down
Case Mysteries No.5

**Section Nine**
The Stupidity of Nicotine Replacement 'Therapy'
*also,* Marketing, Slander and Excuses:
i). The Promotion of a Poison
ii). Peddling Doubt
iii). Beggaring Belief

**Section Ten**
The Compulsive Habit Structure
Case Mysteries No.6
A Pause for Breath

That first Volume is still available on Amazon and at least another dozen on-line booksellers. There should be more books following later – shorter ones! - including one about weight loss with hypnotherapy, also some interesting stuff about hypnotherapy and gambling, alcohol and drugs, phobias... I'll try to make it all entertaining as well as informative and (I hope) genuinely useful. Bye for now!

CPSIA information can be obtained at www.ICGtesting.com
Printed in the USA
LVOW061650210212
269754LV00002B/25/P